AMERICAN RED CROSS

HOME NURSING
TEXTBOOK

AMERICAN RED CROSS

HOME NURSING
TEXTBOOK

PREPARED
UNDER THE SUPERVISION OF
NURSING SERVICES, AMERICAN RED CROSS

1950
THE BLAKISTON COMPANY
PHILADELPHIA

PRINTED IN THE U. S. A., BY J. W CLEMENT CO., BUFFALO, N. Y.

ABOUT THIS BOOK

NEARLY every family has an illness or injury some time; much of the worry and confusion that often results can be reduced if some member of the family has the knowledge and skill required to give simple home nursing care to the sick or injured.

Increasingly, doctors are recommending home rather than hospital care for many patients if conditions are favorable. This is especially true when constant attendance by an expert or the use of specialized equipment are not needed. Individual, personalized, loving service in a familiar environment—the home—plays an important role in the recovery of the patient.

The instruction given in this book assumes that the patient's treatments, other than emergency first aid, are ordered by a physician and that the general nursing care is under a doctor's supervision or that of a professional registered nurse.

Many times the home nurse's skill in carrying out the treatments ordered by the doctor will shorten an illness, and her ability to keep a patient comfortable will make the whole experience less disturbing to the patient and to the household. The doctor will find that an intelligent, orderly report of his patient's condition and the care given by the home nurse under his direction will be helpful in making a diagnosis of the illness, in prescribing for it, and in judging its progress. When some member of the family knows how to recognize signs of illness, how to protect others from infection, and how to give simple nursing care, serious complications may be avoided, the disease shortened or prevented from spreading to others, and the patient made more comfortable. As a general rule, the homemaker has the responsibility for giving care to the sick at home and should, therefore, be able to give it as effectively as possible. However, other members of the family can also profit from this instruction, as there is frequently a need to share the responsibility to prevent it from becoming too heavy a burden for one person to carry. Also, the homemaker may herself be the patient, in which case some other member of the family would be forced to assume the responsibility.

Home nursing instruction is of special value to young people of high school age and older, since it not only prepares them to give direct assistance in the event that someone in the family is ill but also gives them a better understanding of the special needs in caring for the sick and prepares them for the future when they themselves will be homemakers. It also frequently serves as an introduction to nursing as a profession they would like to follow.

There is art as well as skill in giving nursing care, and the welfare of the patient is usually as dependent upon the spirit in which care is given as upon the skill employed.

This book, prepared primarily as a textbook for those who take the Red Cross Home Nursing Course, will help the home nurse learn:

1. How to meet simple home emergencies.
2. How to recognize some of the early signs of illness.
3. How to give simple nursing care to the sick and injured at home.
4. How to help keep the family well.

The book provides detailed instructions for carrying out many home nursing procedures and includes selected additional references for those who wish to study further.

FOREWORD

THIS IS the sixth revision of the official Red Cross textbook on home nursing that has been issued under various titles since the publication of *Elementary Hygiene and Care of the Sick,* prepared by Jane A. Delano and Isabel McIsaac, in 1913. The home nursing program of the Red Cross is based on the premise that family health protection and home care of the sick are essentially a family concern, and that homemakers and potential homemakers need to have the skills and knowledge that enable them to carry such responsibility effectively. These textbooks have provided a guide for over 3,000,000 individuals who have completed the Red Cross Home Nursing Course, and for innumerable others who want a source of ready reference on home care of the sick.

Nursing Services of the American National Red Cross acknowledge with deep appreciation the invaluable contributions made by the many persons who have shared in the preparation of this book. We regret that it is impossible to list each individual by name.

Our special gratitude is extended to Dorothy Deming for her untiring effort in assembling the content of the book, and to representatives of the professional staff of the Public Health Service and the Children's Bureau of the Federal Security Agency, the Advisory Board on Health Services of the American Red Cross, and the Joint Orthopedic Nursing Advisory Service for their critical review of the scientific content and for their assistance in the preparation of material. To Bartholomew Valosio, the Red Cross Photographic Laboratory, and the U. S. Department of Agriculture for the illustrations; to the administrative and technical staff of other Red Cross Services for their review of the manuscript and their valuable suggestions; and last, but not least, to our faithful clerical staff, we express our appreciation.

RUTH B. FREEMAN,
Administrator, Nursing Services

CONTENTS

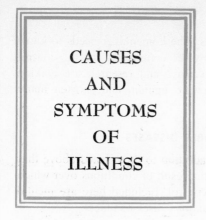

CAUSES
AND
SYMPTOMS
OF
ILLNESS

1

DISEASES may generally be classed as communicable (catching) or non-communicable. They vary in their severity and consequences. Sometimes a disease may be entirely unnoticed until it has made significant progress. Transfer of infection is possible in the early stages of communicable disease. Consequently, if there is a question concerning the nature of an illness it should be considered communicable until its identity is known.

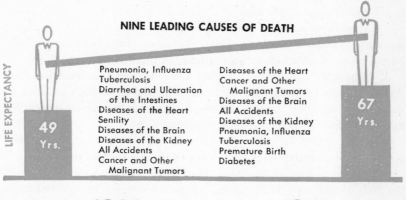

NINE LEADING CAUSES OF DEATH

LIFE EXPECTANCY

1900	1947
49 Yrs.	67 Yrs.

1900:
Pneumonia, Influenza
Tuberculosis
Diarrhea and Ulceration of the Intestines
Diseases of the Heart
Senility
Diseases of the Brain
Diseases of the Kidney
All Accidents
Cancer and Other Malignant Tumors

1947:
Diseases of the Heart
Cancer and Other Malignant Tumors
Diseases of the Brain
All Accidents
Diseases of the Kidney
Pneumonia, Influenza
Tuberculosis
Premature Birth
Diabetes

In the United States in 1947, the nine leading causes of death in the order of their occurrence were heart diseases, cancer, cerebral hemorrhage, accidents, diseases of the kidneys, pneumonia, tuberculosis, premature birth, and diabetes.[1] These causes of death, however, are not necessarily the most frequent causes of illness. With the exception of pneumonia and tuberculosis, the diseases listed above are not classed as

[1] *United States Summary of Vital Statistics, 1947:* Vital Statistics—Special Reports, State Summaries, **30**:7 (Sept. 15, 1949), Public Health Service, Federal Security Agency, Washington, D. C.

1

communicable; yet they are all perilous. The homemaker needs to know about and use the facilities provided by the community for the control and care of illness. Modern medical science and research are making great progress in learning how to prevent, lighten, and shorten many dangerous diseases.

NONCOMMUNICABLE DISEASES

There are a great many diseases in addition to those listed above that are noncommunicable. These may be the result of conditions over which the individual may or may not have control. Included here are mental diseases, which today are one of the major causes of illness.

Some conditions leading to the development of noncommunicable diseases are:

1. An inborn defect in one of the organs or systems of the body. Such a condition may run in the family. A person faced with a constitutional weakness such as a tendency to have diabetes can plan living and working habits that will protect these organs or systems from any unnecessary strain and thus, perhaps, avoid a chronic disability.

2. A previous attack of some acute communicable disease leading to a noncommunicable condition. Heart disease in adults, for example, may be the result of an attack of scarlet fever or diphtheria in childhood.

3. Longtime exposure to irritating substances or continued irritation on any part of the body. Exposure to industrial dusts such as silica or quartz, for example, damages the lungs and makes the person susceptible to chronic diseases of the lung or to tuberculosis.

4. Faulty living habits, particularly in relation to food, drugs, and rest. Lack of essential foods may lead to a disease such as scurvy.

5. Failure to have proper medical attention until the affected part of the body becomes so badly damaged that it can never be restored to its normal condition or function. Perhaps the best example of such neglect is fatal cancer resulting from disregard of a painless, tiny lump or thickening, especially in the breast, or any sore that does not heal, particularly on the lip or tongue.

6. The aging process, with its accompanying changes in the body, may lead to illness; for example, circulation tends to slow down and the individual may become more susceptible to upper respiratory infection (infection in the upper breathing tract, including the nose and throat) because of lessened blood supply.

Measures for preventing the development of noncommunicable diseases are:

1. Observance of healthful living habits.
2. Routine checkup by a doctor.
3. Prompt reporting to the doctor of any symptoms of illness.
4. Bed rest, if ill, until the doctor gives his diagnosis and orders and until he gives his permission to resume usual activities.

Mental Illness. Mental illness is one of the chief health problems today. Its importance is indicated by the fact that there are about as many patients in the hospitals for the mentally ill as in all other hospitals combined. Outside the mental hospitals also are many persons incapable of living normal, useful lives because they are suffering various degrees of emotional disturbance.

The prevention of mental illness depends upon medical research, which will help us learn the health education and supportive measures that will promote mental health and happiness, just as we have been able to do in the field of physical illness. It will depend also upon recognition that much of the groundwork for mental disease is laid in early childhood. Thus, all measures taken by individuals and community groups to encourage congenial and healthy family life will help prevent future breakdowns. In addition, the community must be willing to support measures that will assist in preparing professional people to be more skilled in the knowledge of mental health, prevention of mental illness, and early recognition of behavior disorders. This means that community leaders must know what modern treatment for mental illness is and be willing to pay for such treatment.

Fortunately, every year more is learned about the steps to take to prevent mental illness. We know that all people need a sense of security and belonging, a feeling of individual worth, and an opportunity to be prepared for a vocation of their choice. They need an inner sense of security, which comes from developing a balance between their own individual desires and the limitations of the social group in which they live. Prevention, therefore, takes the form of providing security, love, companionship, and wholesome recreation for children; vocational and personal guidance into the right kind of job for the adolescent; and marriage counseling, homemaking, job interest, economic security, and constructive recreation for the adult. Excessive worry, overwork, unhappy marriages, and ill health may be steps in a series of incidents that contribute to mental breakdowns.

Individuals and families in many progressive communities will find numerous resources to help them build protective walls against some of the conditions that threaten mental health. Probably the most important

first step in preventing mental illness is to share the trouble with an
understanding and wise adviser. The help of family physicians, public
health nurses, psychiatrists (doctors for mental illness), pastors, or some
other wise and trusted person should be sought when problems are over-
whelming and one's sense of security or happiness is threatened.

Community organization for preventing mental illness, for the detec-
tion and treatment of the early symptoms of emotional distress, and for
the treatment of the mentally ill person who does not require hospitalization is another essential. The provision of mental hygiene clinics is an
important consideration. These clinics are variously labeled *child guidance clinics, adult counseling clinics, mental hygiene clinics, alcoholic
clinics,* and so on. They sometimes are conducted by voluntary agencies;
more recently they may be óne of the newer services developed by the
department of health in the community. Many communities are today
sponsoring citizen participation in mental hygiene societies that are active
in the planning and promotion of all types of mental health and treatment resources.

Some important things to remember about mental illnesses are:

1. The practice of mental health begins in the home—*every* home.

2. Counsel and treatment from experts in the mental health field
should be sought at once when tensions and undesirable behavior begin to
appear. Medical care is most successful when the patient seeks help early.

3. Symptoms begin slowly and may not be evident for some time, and
a long time may be needed to cure mental illness.

4. Community resources should be used. These should be varied
enough to care for the periods when strains are liable to develop. Every
community should have access to services that will assist:

   a. Parents to care for the emotional as well as the physical needs
      of the baby.
   b. Teachers to guide the developing personality of the child.
   c. Industrial leaders to plan coöperatively with employees for bet-
      ter job adjustment and happier work relationships.
   d. Community leaders to develop sound community health pro-
      grams, mental as well as physical.

"Health is a state of complete physical, mental, and social well-being
and not merely the absence of disease or infirmity."[2] With the recent
advances of modern medicine and education, the opportunities for mental health are brighter for the future than ever before in history. The
home nurse can do her part by applying the principles of mental health

---

[2] From the Preamble to the Constitution of the World Health Organization.

in her own home, by participating actively in community mental health organizations, and by helping people accept the use of psychiatrists, mental health clinics, and other resources for treatment.

COMMUNICABLE DISEASES

A communicable disease, briefly, is a disease that can be transmitted from human or animal hosts to susceptible individuals. The means of transfer depends upon the disease. It may be direct through contact with a sick person's infected discharges, such as droplets coughed or breathed, or indirect through such means as contaminated (soiled by contact with infectious material) water or food, or insects.

It is important to understand a few terms that the doctor and professional nurse will use in speaking of communicable diseases. Some of these are:

1. *Infection:* This refers to the condition in which harmful organisms grow and multiply in the body. It may also refer to the communication of disease from one person to another either by direct contact or by contact with some body discharge.

2. *Incubation period:* This is the time that elapses between the original infection of a susceptible person with the disease germs and the appearance of the symptoms of the disease.

3. *Communicable period:* The length of time during which the disease is transferable to another person.

4. *Contamination:* The presence of infectious material in or on any object. A *person* is infected; an *object* is contaminated.

5. *Isolation:* The separation of the infected person from others so that the spread of his disease to others is prevented.

6. *Disinfection:* Destroying or getting rid of the germs. (Sterilization— killing germs by means of heat—is one form of disinfection.) When all the discharges and contaminated objects are disinfected routinely during a patient's illness, the process is called *concurrent* disinfection. When everything is disinfected and cleaned after the illness, the procedure is known as *terminal* disinfection. In many communicable diseases both are necessary. The attending physician or local health department will advise regarding safe methods of disinfection.

7. *Quarantine:* Limiting the freedom of persons ill with or exposed to a communicable disease so they cannot go about among others and possibly give them the disease. The period varies with the type of disease and usually is determined by health department regulations. Sometimes the entire family is so limited or quarantined. Try to become

acquainted with local health department regulations governing such quarantine, as they vary considerably in certain respects in different sections of the country.

8. *Placarding:* The official posting by the health department of a notice upon a house indicating that a communicable disease is present. Many communities have discontinued this practice for almost all diseases.

9. *Carrier:* One who is able to transfer his disease to another susceptible person without showing symptoms of the disease himself.

The doctor, the local health department, the Visiting Nurse Association, and the school or industry where members of the family go are all interested in helping avoid communicable diseases. If every citizen reports symptoms of illness promptly, takes all possible means to prevent and control the spread of communicable diseases, and obeys the doctor's order to the letter, a large portion of the cases reported every year in this country can be prevented.

Microörganisms

Everywhere—in the air, water, and ground, in plants and animals, and even in our own bodies—are tiny forms of life that can be seen only through the powerful lens of a microscope. Scientists have given these organisms the general names of bacteria, protozoa, fungi, and viruses. Some of these organisms are definitely helpful to human life. Examples of such organisms are the bacteria that help keep the soil fertile so that it grows better crops, the bacteria in yeast that make bread rise, and the bacteria used in making vinegar. However, the harmful microörganisms usually referred to as disease germs are among the worst enemies of man because they are responsible for many of the diseases of both men and animals.

Most communicable diseases are caused by germs that enter through the body openings, particularly the nose and throat. Some of these organisms, however, get into the body through a break in the skin or membrane and attack the tissues at that point. Then the body defenses come to the rescue, and, if they stop further action of these organisms, we say infection is localized. If the body defenses are not able to stop further action and the tiny organisms get into the blood stream and travel to all parts of the body, a condition of general infection sometimes called blood poisoning ensues. If the attack is light and can be quickly overcome, the illness does not last long. But if the germs are especially vigorous and the body defenses have a hard time in controlling them, a long and severe illness may follow. When the body is unable to make the proper defense, with or without outside help, we lose the fight and death results. If it were not for the fact that the organisms of most human infections die soon after they leave the body of the infected person, unless they immediately find another host (susceptible person), they would have destroyed the human race long ago.

Protection Against Disease-producing Germs

Natural Resistance. The human being is not susceptible to some diseases caused by organisms that affect other animals, as the human body does not provide the proper soil conditions for growth. The resistance that man has to these diseases is called natural resistance.

The newborn child may be immune for some time after birth to some diseases, depending in part on whether the mother herself is resistant to the disease.

Doctors usually advise that children be protected against smallpox, diphtheria, and whooping cough during their first year of life because any natural resistance is lost after about the sixth month.

Acquired Resistance. Another kind of resistance or protection is developed by frequent exposure to disease germs or by exposure to small numbers of germs over a long period of time. This is the kind of resistance some adults have built up against diseases that are common among children.

It is well known that people develop resistance to some diseases by having the disease itself. This resistance may be apparent for a very short period or last a lifetime. An attack of typhoid fever, whooping cough, or smallpox usually makes an individual immune to that disease for life, although second attacks are reported occasionally.

Artificial Protection. Another way to obtain protection against certain communicable diseases is by artificial immunity or protection. Scientists, in addition to discovering how the body defends itself, have discovered ways by which we can bring outside assistance to help the fight against some diseases. Successful vaccination (protective inoculation) of the infant against smallpox, for example, will usually provide protection for several years, but should be repeated as advised by the doctor. As a matter of safety, the child should be vaccinated just before he enters school, whether he has been vaccinated before or not. If a child is immune from a previous vaccination, a revaccination may show a slight skin reaction but will not produce illness. As far as possible, as soon as natural immunity wears off, a person should be protected by artificial immunity

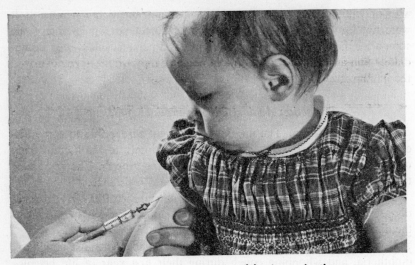

Many diseases can be prevented by immunization.

from those communicable diseases for which we have an immunizing agent and to which he is most likely to be exposed.

Some of the diseases for which we have protection if proper immunization is carried out are noted in the chart at the back of this book. The chart also lists some diseases whose attack can be lightened and shortened by giving the body additional help in fighting the germs already there. Because more and more is discovered each year about protection from infections of all types, any chart printed today may be out of date tomorrow. Therefore, ask the doctor about immunization.

Transmitting Infection

Germs may enter the body directly by way of contaminated water or foods; they may be breathed in with air containing germ-laden dust; or they may enter through contact with material contaminated by the body's discharges, which accumulate on such articles as soiled handkerchiefs. Every communicable disease comes from a person, insect, or other animal capable of spreading the infection directly or indirectly. The discharges of the nose, mouth, genital organs, and occasionally the bowels and bladder, or open sores may contain the germs. The blood may also contain germs. Milk that has not been pasteurized or boiled may transfer such diseases as undulant fever or tuberculosis; the bite of an infected flea may cause plague; the sting of an infected mosquito may cause malaria. Infection also may be transferred by a human carrier, a well person who carries the germs of a disease in his body but who is without signs of having the disease himself. Such a person may have had the disease at some previous time and recovered or may be suffering from a mild form of the disease without having the characteristic symptoms. The diseases most often carried in this way are diphtheria, scarlet fever, and typhoid fever, but there are others. The carrier serves as a host to undesirable germs that have taken up temporary or permanent residence within his body and are harmless to him because his body defenses are able to keep them under control. Carriers have been known to harbor germs of typhoid fever for many years.

Protection Through Clean Habits. Since disease germs can live indefinitely in the mucous membranes (lining of the body cavities that open to the outside of the body) of the nose and throat or in the intestinal tract of healthy people, but may be harmful if transferred to others, all of us should consider ourselves possible carriers and develop habits that will protect us and our associates. Young children and sick or aged people, who may not have the ability to resist disease, are especially in need of protection. Clean habits are more than good manners; they are an obligation to one's family and one's community.

Coughing and Sneezing. When a person coughs or sneezes and sprays the discharges from his nose and throat into the air, or even when he talks and laughs, tiny droplets of saliva (spittle) are thrown out to fall where they may. If another person is close enough to receive these droplets, he may become infected by some germ that the person has been harboring. Some germs die quickly when exposed to light and air. Others may live for some time in the droplet, even after it dries. To protect others, one should hold a handkerchief or tissue over both the nose *and* mouth when sneezing or coughing. If the sneeze comes unexpectedly before protection of the mouth and nose is possible, one should turn the head away from other people. A person should not stand close to another person's face when laughing or talking; spray from an explosive sneeze or laugh may carry 6 or 8 feet; it cannot be escaped at 12 inches. Coughing and sneezing are among the worst offenders in the spread of communicable diseases.

Because the hands are in frequent contact with your nose and mouth, they are often a means of carrying germs from one person to another.

Other methods of transmission are using another person's drinking cup, eating with the same fork or spoon, biting from the same apple, sucking the same lollipop, and kissing. These routes are especially dangerous to small children, because they do not have ways of protecting themselves from careless older people.

General Precautions. As a protection against communicable diseases, one should practice these rules:

1. Avoid contact with people who are suffering from communicable diseases.

2. Anyone with a cold, discharging nose, or cough should use paper handkerchiefs or clean soft rags that may be used once and then tucked into a paper bag and destroyed without further handling. The nose and mouth should be covered when sneezing or coughing.

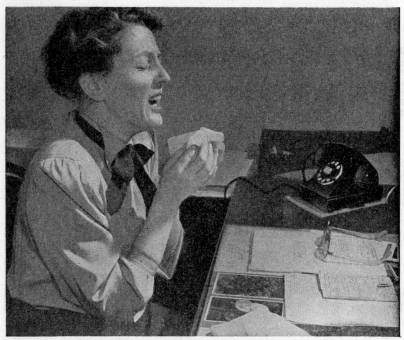

Catch that first sneeze! Protect others from infection.

3. Keep the fingers away from the face, mouth, and eyes.

4. Keep all soiled articles such as pencils, pins, and money out of the mouth.

5. Avoid raising dust when cleaning the floors, especially when food is exposed.

6. Always wash the hands before eating, before preparing food, after handling contaminated articles, and after going to the toilet. Wash the

hands after caring for a sick person or handling pets. (*See* Washing the Hands, p. 139.)

7. Keep personal articles clean and reserve for personal use only.

8. Use safe water, milk, and other food supplies. Keep milk and other perishable foods under refrigeration when possible.

9. Always use clean glasses, cups, plates, or other eating utensils at home, and keep the fingers off the parts of dishes or silverware that will touch the lips. Try to frequent only those restaurants, food counters, or stores where the cooks and servers are under good supervision, and where the service and utensils are known to be clean.

10. Keep the general health at a high level by eating the right kind and quantity of food and by getting an adequate amount of sleep, rest, sunshine, fresh air, and exercise.

11. Obtain from the doctor protection from the diseases for which there are immunizing agents and to which one may be exposed.

12. Look with suspicion on any illness that starts with headache, fever, nausea, sore throat, running eyes or nose, stiff neck, sneezing, aching, and a general feeling of being "all in." Anyone feeling that way should try to keep away from others, go to bed if possible, and call the doctor if symptoms persist. As a safety measure, use paper tissues for discharges from the nose and throat, destroy them after use, and be sure that the dishes are washed in hot soapsuds and rinsed with scalding water.

How To Kill Germs

Fortunately, there are many ways of destroying germs. Some germs die quickly on exposure to sunlight and thorough drying; others are so hardy that high temperatures are needed to kill them. When we kill all the germs present on an object, such as a compress or dressing pad for a wound, we say we sterilize it. Hospitals have special sterilizers for this purpose.

In the home the spread of infection may be prevented by various methods such as burning, boiling, scalding, sunning articles, or using chemicals, as ordered by the doctor. The most common method of getting rid of germs on contaminated articles is to wash them thoroughly with hot soapy water, rinsing well, and, if the material can stand it, scalding and allowing to drain dry. The hands, which cannot stand scalding, need extra time and rubbing to make them as clean as possible.

If an infectious condition is present in which germs do not die easily, the doctor will give instructions as to the care of articles in contact with the patient as well as how to disinfect the discharges from the body.

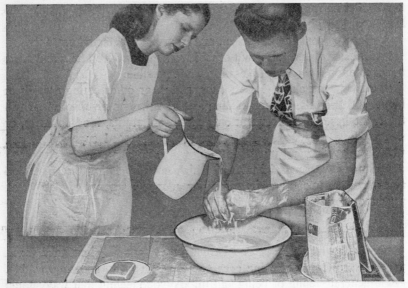

Cleanliness lessens spread of infection to and from patient.

The home nurse can always assume that germs are present in discharges from the nose, mouth, throat, bowels, urinary bladder, genitals, and any discharging surface. She should cleanse *everything* in contact with such discharges, including the hands. This is a wise precaution in all illness.

SYMPTOMS OF PHYSICAL ILLNESS

Some of the symptoms described here may be evident only to the sufferer, while others may be evident only to someone else. Babies and small children are not able to describe their feelings, and mothers must learn to recognize the location of pain or discomfort in the child by his behavior. Many signs of illness can be detected only by scientific apparatus in the hands of a skilled doctor or laboratory technician, and even these are not always sufficient to determine the diagnosis. The results of tests must be studied along with the complaints of the sick person, the history of his past illnesses, and the reports of the person who takes care of him. Finally, in making his diagnosis the doctor sometimes depends as much on the absence of certain signs as on the presence of others.

For all these reasons, the keen observation of symptoms is important for the home nurse. Furthermore, frequently the earlier the symptoms are noticed and the sufferer placed under medical care, the more rapid will be his recovery. The symptoms described here are not listed in the order of their frequency or importance, because each person differs in his reactions to illness. Nor is the severity of a symptom a true guide to its importance. Even a mild symptom may be a forerunner of serious illness.

Children and many adults who know that their physical condition is being carefully watched are likely to exaggerate every little ache or pain. Usually they do not intend to mislead. Often such exaggeration is simply an unconscious attempt to get satisfaction from special attention. In any case, observe symptoms without the person's knowledge as far as possible, and without too much obvious concern, so that his interest or anxiety may not be especially excited.

Symptoms of physical and mental illness are seldom separable, but for clarity they are presented separately here.

Appearance

The Face. The appearance of the face often gives a clue to the nature of an illness and to how much the patient is actually suffering. The facial expression is sometimes drawn and haggard, or it may be alert and anxious, or dull and listless. The face may seem swollen or puffy about the eyes; it may be flushed or pale.

The eyes may seem heavy or unusually bright. Note whether they show any evidence of inflammation (diseased condition of the body tissue resulting in redness, swelling, heat, and pain) or discharge or whether they appear bloodshot or unusually sensitive to light. Some diseases are characterized by disturbance of vision; the doctor should be told if the patient complains of spots before the eyes, of "halos" around lights, of seeing double, or of not being able to see clearly.

If the whites of the eyes are yellow or show a yellowish tinge, report the condition to the physician.

Any unusual condition noted in the eye itself, such as crossed eyes or difficulty in seeing objects, should receive attention from a physician. (*See* Putting Drops in the Eyes, p. 196.)

The Nose and Throat. Bleeding or other discharge or difficulty in breathing and swallowing should be noted.

A running nose, sneezing, coughing, hoarseness, difficulty in breathing, and sore throat are all symptoms of the common cold. They may also mean the onset of grippe, influenza, pneumonia, bronchitis, laryngitis, sinusitis—in fact, any abnormality of the respiratory tract. All these symptoms, especially when accompanied by fever, should be reported to the doctor, and any one of them that persists should be a matter of grave concern and should be given medical attention. A chronic (of long duration) cough, chronic hoarseness, and continued difficulty in breathing are especially serious.

The Mouth. The gums in health are pink and firm, but in illness they may be swollen, bleeding, and sensitive. In illness the tongue may be dry and cracked, or have a heavy white or yellowish coating, or may be a vivid red and have a raw appearance; when extended it may tremble noticeably. The sense of taste is nearly always disturbed, especially when there is a high temperature or difficulty in breathing through the nose.

The Voice. The voice is often changed in sickness; it may be weak, hoarse, or whispering. In extreme weakness speech may be difficult. Any unusual moaning, groaning, and crying should be noted as an indication of some disturbance.

The Skin. The skin of the whole body should be observed for discoloration, swelling, itching, rash, or eruptions of any kind. Sometimes there is puffiness of the skin under the eyes, or swelling around the wrists or ankles. Any of these symptoms should be reported to the doctor.

Appetite

Loss of appetite usually accompanies illness. Therefore the amount and kind of food eaten should be recorded for the doctor, as well as the amount of water or other liquids taken.

Occasionally, sick people have strong cravings for certain foods or will develop enormous appetites. Children may eat unusual things such as dirt, plaster, or grass. Any unusual food habit should be reported to the doctor.

Weight

Continued loss of weight in either adults or children is usually a sign that something is wrong. It may be caused by disease, disordered function of the internal organs, mental distress, or insufficient or the wrong type of food. A definite gain in weight may also indicate a change in condition. Nearly everyone loses weight in a severe illness; therefore, it is of special importance for the home nurse to provide nourishing foods to protect the body from too great a weight loss.

Persons over 40 years of age will find it to their advantage to be short a few pounds rather than burdened with an excess of weight. Statistics show that the incidence of heart disease or diabetes is higher in overweight people. Too much weight is also a handicap to activity and good posture. It often leads to trouble with the feet because the arches are strained from carrying too heavy a load.

Sleep

The number of hours a patient sleeps should be recorded as accurately as possible. The word of the patient on this subject is not always reliable, however. When ill, a short period of wakefulness may seem much longer than it really is, especially at night. It should be noted whether sleep is quiet or restless and whether the patient sleeps in short naps or for a long time.

A person in bed all the time may not need as much sleep as when he is up and about, but remember that sleep is nature's way of resting the mind and body and is one of the essential "medicines." The home nurse should make every effort to give her patient long periods of rest and sleep and should insist on daytime naps for the convalescent patient (one who is in process of gradual restoration to health), the young, and the old.

General Malaise (Indefinite Feeling of Discomfort) or Weakness

A feeling of general discomfort, weakness, and fatigue—of being too weary to move—may be present at the beginning of an illness and usually accompanies early convalescence after a serious illness. At the start of an illness, such symptoms may be combined with headache, sore throat, and fever. In children illness is shown by irritability, poor posture, and lack of interest in play. Persistent fatigue in the morning may indicate the inability of the body to benefit by rest periods.

Fever

Feeling chilly, alternating with feeling hot, may mean fever. The skin may be dry and hot. Usually some loss of appetite, considerable thirst, and general discomfort accompany fever.

Fever is a sign that something is out of order in the body, although sometimes a person may be ill but still be without fever. A change from the normal body temperature has been used by doctors for years in judging whether a person is sick, in diagnosing and treating illness, and in noting the stages of recovery. One of the first questions when sickness strikes will be: "What is the temperature?" Therefore, it is desirable that each household own and know how to use a clinical thermometer and know what to report to the doctor. (*See* Taking the Temperature, p. 141.)

The temperature usually is taken by mouth, although it may also be taken by rectum or in the armpit. For infants, very young children, and unconscious or very ill patients, or for those unable to keep the lips closed, the temperature should be taken by rectum or armpit.

When To Take the Temperature. The home nurse should take the temperature:

1. Whenever a person complains of feeling ill or shows signs of illness.

2. During illness, once or twice a day at the same time each day, usually in the morning and afternoon, or as the doctor orders, which may be three or four times a day or only once a week, depending on the condition and age of the patient.

3. Whenever there is a sudden change in the patient's condition, such as a chill, restlessness, or pain.

4. Whenever there is headache, pain in the chest or abdomen, sore throat, chills, vomiting, diarrhea (frequent watery or slimy stools), or skin rash.

These symptoms may mean the presence of serious illness or of conditions needing immediate medical or surgical attention. A person with a head cold or cough with a mouth temperature of over 99.6°F. (Fahrenheit) should not go to work or school but should remain at home away from others, preferably in bed. A higher temperature together with other symptoms indicates the need of medical care.

It is unnecessary to wake a patient for the purpose of taking his temperature at a specific time unless the doctor has requested it. Do not take the temperature immediately after the patient has had a hot or cold bath, hot or cold food or drink, or has been smoking. Do not take a rectal temperature immediately after an enema or when the rectum is full of fecal matter (bowel content). The local temperature registered may not then be the true temperature of the whole body.

Pulse and Respiration

The pulse rate, even with persons in good health, varies with the individual. Age and sex account for some of these variations. A child's pulse rate, for example, is faster than that of an adult; a woman's pulse rate is usually faster than that of a man. While there are great variations, the rate for a man is about 70 beats each minute, and for a woman from 75 to 80 beats each minute. The rate for children varies greatly. As a rule the pulse rate increases with a rise in temperature, although this is not always true.

The pulse may be felt most easily where a large artery is near the surface; this may be on the inside of the wrist, at the ankle, or at the temple. The inner side of the wrist below the thumb is the place most often used to record the pulse because it is usually the most convenient.

The pulse should be counted after the patient has been resting quietly, or in a child when asleep. The beat of the pulse is usually as regular as the ticking of a clock. Any irregularity should be called to the doctor's attention. A watch with a second hand will be helpful in counting. (*See* Taking the Pulse and Respiration, p. 146.)

Respiration or breathing is also usually faster when a person has a fever. Because the rate of breathing can be controlled to some extent by the patient, the count should be made when the patient is unaware that it is being taken. In addition to the count, the doctor will want to know about anything unusual, such as difficult and painful breathing.

Pain

Pain is an important sign in illness and should never be disregarded. *Pain is nature's warning that something is wrong.* Pain cannot be measured; therefore, we must rely entirely on the patient's description of it. Some patients overemphasize minor pains and others disregard severe ones. The doctor must draw his own conclusions, after considering all other symptoms in relation to the pain. Frequently the alert home nurse has come to know the patient's habitual responses to pain and is in a good position to judge their nature. The facts to be reported to the doctor are: the location and duration of the pain; when it is most severe; whether it is relieved or increased by a change of position, eating, or drinking; and the patient's description of the pain as dull or sharp, stabbing, throbbing, or continuous, slight or severe.

Abdominal Pain and Stomach-ache. Pain in the abdomen or stomach may be caused by improper eating or food poisoning, or it may be due to appendicitis or some other acute and serious condition in the abdomen. Abdominal pain caused by poisoning from spoiled or unclean food is often accompanied by diarrhea and vomiting. Typhoid fever may also start with abdominal pain and diarrhea. If a stomach-ache is not relieved by rest and withholding food, report this to the doctor. *Do not give a laxative. Do not give an enema.*

There are so many possibilities that abdominal pain may be serious that the doctor should be notified and the condition treated with great care.

Chest Pain. Pain in the chest is serious, especially if accompanied by fever, coughing, or difficulty in breathing. Make the patient comfortable in bed, propped against pillows if that eases the pain, and send for the doctor at once.

Headache. Headache is a symptom common to many diseases and disorders. It may be caused by eyestrain, constipation, indigestion, infection,

fatigue, lack of sleep, or some other disorder. To treat a headache effectively, the cause should be determined first. Before taking any home remedy, one should ask oneself whether a little less food, or a little more sleep,
exercise, fresh air, or drinking water might not relieve the condition. Some
people have severe reactions from drugs that are common home remedies.
Frequent headaches require a doctor's advice; a sharp, sudden headache
that continues should be reported to the doctor at once. To postpone this
only causes needless suffering and delays diagnosis and treatment.

Sore Throat. Sore throats are of many varieties and the result of many
conditions, the most usual type being an inflamed, raw throat, with or
without whitish patches, caused by an infection. Sore throats accompany

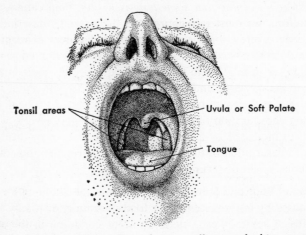

Tonsil areas

Uvula or Soft Palate

Tongue

Look in back and sides of throat for redness, swelling, and white or gray spots.

many communicable diseases and may be present during colds, coughs,
some stomach upsets, and fever. They may be caused by infected tonsils.
Difficulty and pain in swallowing are the usual symptoms. Severe sore and
swollen throats, or painful throat conditions that continue, with fever, or
throats that show yellow patches, grayish patches, or are very raw and
bleeding should be reported to the doctor immediately. Throat symptoms
are important in diagnosing several of the communicable diseases.

All patients with sore throats should keep away from others, go to bed
if there is fever or if there are any patches on the throat, have separate
service from the rest of the family (*see* The Patient with a Communicable
Disease, p. 67), drink plenty of water, and eat only a light or liquid diet.
(*See* Standard Diets Usually Ordered by Doctors, Table 1, p. 58.)

So many of the early signs of illness include a sore throat that it is desirable not only to learn how to inspect a throat easily, quickly, and skillfully, but also to accustom children to opening their mouths and saying "ah." If this inspection is made a frequent routine when a child is well, he will not object to having his throat inspected when he is sick and it will be much easier for the home nurse to do this. (*See* Inspecting the Throat, p. 187.)

Earache. Any discharges from the ears or any pain, tenderness, or swelling about the ears should be reported to the doctor at once. Also report complaints of the patient about pain or crackling in the ears when swallowing. Sometimes the hearing is affected, even though outward evidence of trouble in the ears is lacking. (*See* Foreign Bodies, In the Ear, p. 97.)

Backache. There are so many causes of backache—some of them serious—that a doctor should be consulted if the pain persists.

Stiff Neck. A stiff neck is sometimes a symptom of serious illness. *Report to the doctor at once* if it is accompanied by fever, vomiting, or sore throat or if the head is held back rigidly. If the cause appears to be muscular strain, heat may be applied. A stiff neck may be a more serious symptom in children than in adults.

Nausea and Vomiting

If nausea and vomiting are accompanied by severe cramps or abdominal pain, they should be reported to the doctor, as they may be symptoms of appendicitis. Vomiting, if caused by indigestion, usually brings its own relief. The color, general appearance, and amount of material vomited should be observed. If vomiting is continuous, severe, accompanied by blood or dark material, or has an offensive odor, report this to the doctor and save the vomitus for him to see.

Bowel Movements

In sickness the number and nature of the bowel movements and their color and consistency should be noted. The normal color is brown or yellow and the consistency somewhat soft. If there is any difference from this, a stool (bowel movement) should be saved for the doctor to see. The bowel movement in typhoid fever and some forms of dysentery harbors disease germs that are positive evidence of the nature of the disease. In such cases the doctor will give directions for the safe disposal of body wastes.

Constipation. Normally, foods in the process of digestion pass through the intestines and out of the lower bowel as waste matter (the stool or feces) once in 24 to 36 hours. If the right foods are eaten in the right amount and if plenty of water is taken, the bowel habits usually become regular and elimination takes place—usually after breakfast. When this process is sluggish, the condition is called constipation. Authorities are agreed that the greatest single factor in preventing constipation at any age is the *habit* of evacuating the bowel at a regular time each day. Secondary to habit is the intake of proper food. Conscientious effort should be made to establish a regular time for the bowel movement. Other relief measures may be:

1. One or two glasses of hot or cold water on rising.
2. Drinking more water and fruit juices during the day.
3. Taking special exercise prescribed by the doctor.

Laxatives and enemas are not cures for constipation. A drug taken for the relief of constipation offers only temporary help and frequently does much harm. The intestinal muscles, like all others, must be given an opportunity for natural exercise if they are to be kept in a state of health. When drugs do their work for them, they become weak and flabby. The intelligent way to attack the problems of constipation is to remove the cause by improving the habits. If this fails, a doctor should be consulted.

Diarrhea. Diarrhea (frequent watery or slimy stools) may be caused by an infection, poisonous or undigested food, or emotional strain. In babies or small children, it is usually the result of improper feeding or of unclean water, milk, or other food. It may have serious results. Diarrhea is nature's effort to remove the substances that do not agree with us after they have passed from the stomach into the intestines; it is the natural way of getting rid of poison. Severe or prolonged diarrhea should be reported to the family doctor. Widespread epidemics of sickness have been prevented by a prompt report of such cases. First relief measures for both children and adults in severe cases is to withhold food and give only boiled water until a diagnosis can be made and measures taken to bring relief. After the diarrhea has stopped, a warm liquid or soft diet should be given until the bowel action is regular again. The patient should be kept in bed and kept warm and quiet.

Urination

Inability to urinate (pass or void urine), pain or burning sensations, inability to control the bladder, or too frequent urination should be reported to the doctor. Other points to observe are whether the output is more or less than usual, any change in the usual amber color, and whether there is a deposit of sediment when the urine is left standing. Blood-streaked urine should be reported to the doctor at once.

Painful Menstruation

The discomfort of menstrual pains may often be lessened by good mental hygiene, wholesome living, regular hours, sufficient rest, proper clothing in winter, and protective covering to keep the feet dry in wet weather. Special abdominal exercises prescribed by the doctor and correction of constipation will bring relief sometimes. If improved living habits and relief from worry do not correct the condition, a doctor should be consulted. Some unusual condition in the ovaries or uterus may be responsible for the trouble. Drugs should not be taken except on the advice of the doctor. Relief measures may include rest in bed, hot applications to the feet and back, a hot foot bath, and hot drinks.

If menstruation is accompanied by excessive flowing, or if bleeding occurs between periods, report the matter promptly to a doctor. These may be symptoms of possible cancer.

Discomforts of the Menopause

The cessation of the menstrual periods, which may occur any time after the age of 40—usually around 50—should not be disturbing to the mental and physical health of a woman. There may be uneven intervals between periods, some headache, and occasional days of feeling depressed and blue. The characteristic "hot flashes"—flushing and perspiring that last a few minutes and may occur irregularly over several years—are also usual symptoms and indicate that the body is adjusting itself to the "change of life," which is really a change in the secretions from the endocrine glands (hormones from the ovaries). It is well to keep in touch with the doctor at this time and follow any suggestions he offers for making the changes less troublesome. There are effective medicines to be taken at this time that bring prompt relief, but these must be prescribed by a doctor. Should there be a return of the flow or any bleeding *after the periods have ceased,* the doctor should be consulted promptly.

Men also go through a period of adjustment, usually coming after 50 and before 65, when headaches, depression, backaches, and occasionally frequent urination are present. During this change men should have medical advice. Any enlargement, pain, or discomfort in the region of the prostate gland (discomfort in the lower abdomen and groin) should be reported to the doctor at once.

SYMPTOMS OF MENTAL ILLNESS

The symptoms of mental ill health may be evident to both the sufferer and observer, or possibly neither will recognize them as anything serious. Indeed, mental illness is often so slight that its true symptoms may be exceedingly hard to detect. For this reason and because mental illness calls for tactful and skillful treatment right from the start, the doctor should see the patient when concern is felt for his mental condition. There is no such thing as home first aid for a mental patient if preventive measures have failed. The best help the home nurse can offer is to persuade the patient to see his doctor or a psychiatrist at once.

Some mental conditions accompany illness or result from the use of certain medications and disappear as the patient recovers. Watch carefully the mental condition of a patient who has a high fever, or one who has a severe infection of any kind. When a person is sick, he may become delirious (in a temporary state of mental disturbance) and highly excited, not know where he is, and try to get out of bed; delirious patients should never be left alone.

A disturbed mental condition may be the first sign that a person is physically ill. Confusion in a person's mind about people or events, unreasonable fears, or loss of memory accompany some of the diseased conditions of the glands of the body. Such conditions may disappear entirely with proper treatment.

Undesirable behavior symptoms that should be reported to the doctor if they continue or are frequent are worry, depression, brooding or a feeling that life is useless, inability to concentrate, sleeplessness, headaches not traceable to usual causes, lack of interest in friends, family, job, or play, obsessions (fixed ideas or fears that something is happening or going to happen that is not probable or possible), complaints of an imaginary nature, oversensitivity, reluctance to mingle with others or to go to new places, confusion as to own identity or that of others in the family or as to surroundings, recurrent daydreams or hallucinations (seeing nonexistent objects or having sensations with no external cause) of an impossible nature, and resentment toward one person without apparent cause.

Since the causes of mental illness may be buried deep in past experiences and even then are not always fully understood, treatment must be adjusted to each person. For this reason the psychiatrist or other doctor needs the complete coöperation of the family in whatever line of treatment is chosen.

In many cases only a hospital equipped to care for mental illness can supply the necessary treatment. Often the family find difficulty in accepting this recommendation, but such care may be as essential to the recovery of the patient as is the modern operating room for the safe removal of an infected appendix.

WHAT TO REPORT TO THE DOCTOR

In reporting symptoms to the doctor, the home nurse should be able to tell him the character of the illness, the complaints of the patient, and the symptoms or signs noted, such as:

1. The degree of severity of the pain if any (whether it is a dull ache, acute, or a shooting or stabbing pain), its duration, when it started, its location so far as she can tell, and whether it is concentrated in one place or is influenced by some known behavior, such as eating or the position of the body.

2. The temperature and sometimes the pulse rate. (*See* Taking the Temperature, p. 141, and Taking the Pulse and Respiration, p. 146.)

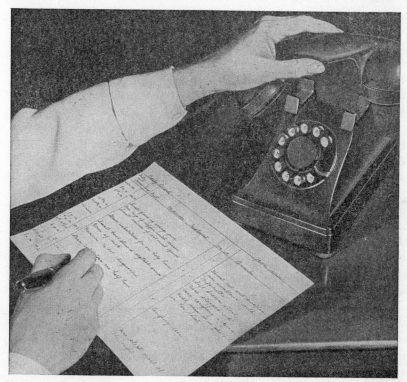

The doctor depends upon accurate and complete reporting by the home nurse.

3. If there is bleeding, its location, color and amount. (*See* Internal Bleeding, p. 90.)

4. The color and character of the stools, vomitus, sputum (spittle) or other discharges (a sample of any discharge of unusual appearance should be saved in a covered container for the doctor to see).

5. A description of the patient's behavior, how he says he feels, and the length of time any undesirable condition has been noticeable.

6. Any other unusual condition noted such as rash, discoloration, or swelling.

7. Any first aid given to relieve the patient.

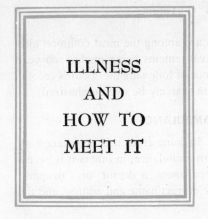

ILLNESS AND HOW TO MEET IT

2

CALLING A DOCTOR

EVERY family should have a doctor to consult regularly for medical advice and treatment. Throughout this book, frequent reference is made to the importance of calling a doctor in time, following his orders exactly, and reporting the progress of the patient to him accurately. Most doctors, unless they know a patient well, prefer not to give medical advice by telephone except in an emergency.

Nearly all counties and cities have a medical society, which is an organization of licensed physicians in good standing. One in doubt about the choice of a doctor, or a newcomer in a community who has not been referred to a doctor there, may ask the medical society to suggest names of local doctors. If there is no medical society, the Visiting Nurse Association, the health department, the local hospital, or a minister may be able to suggest names of doctors. The telephone directory will list local hospitals, health agencies, and the medical society.

Keep the doctor's name and telephone number in a conspicuous place beside the telephone, in the medicine cabinet, on the desk, or in the kitchen, where they can be found easily in an emergency. The entire family should know their location.

If one's regular doctor cannot be reached in an emergency and another is called, the circumstances should be explained to him. This will avoid any misunderstanding when the regular doctor is again available.

Specialists and Consultants

For some illnesses the doctor may wish permission to call in a specialist for consultation, or he may refer the patient to one or to a special clinic. In such an event, it is well to learn in advance what the additional charges will be.

Special Tests

The doctor may recommend special tests if a condition is at all serious, unusual, or uncertain. Many such tests are usually given only in a hospital or a clinic, for example, x-rays, which are among the most common aids to diagnosis. Because of the many advancements being made each year in the diagnosis of disease, the importance of following the doctor's recommendations concerning special tests can scarcely be overemphasized,

CALLING AN AMBULANCE

Find out how to call an ambulance. In some cities it is only necessary to ask the telephone operator to send an ambulance; in others it is necessary to call the hospital, the police department, a doctor, or a druggist. When placing a call, make sure that the correct name and address and the reason for need are given.

In rural areas the ambulance service may be in private hands or community-owned, or there may be none. In the last case a station wagon, truck, or automobile can be converted into an ambulance. For lifting and transporting patients safely, see the *American Red Cross First Aid Textbook,* Chapter 9.

SELECTING A HOSPITAL

When hospital care is necessary, the family doctor will usually suggest the hospital with which he is connected or best acquainted. In a strange community, be sure to select a registered hospital if possible—one approved by the American Hospital Association and the American College of Surgeons. A list of registered hospitals in the community may be obtained from the local medical society, the health department, or the public library.

In addition to general hospitals, special hospitals or divisions of general hospitals provide care for maternity cases, children, orthopedic conditions (deformities), tuberculosis, mental illness, or other conditions.

HEALTH CENTERS AND CLINICS

Health centers and clinics are found in every large city and in nearly all the well-populated rural areas. They may be connected with hospitals as outpatient services (those services provided for persons who are not hospitalized) or with health departments or they may be maintained by some other health agency in the community. Clinics are usually of two types: those where actual treatments are given and those that offer diagnostic and consultant services. Charges may or may not be made for services given. To find out what clinic services are available in a community and their charges, if any, call the local health department, Visiting Nurse Association, or hospital.

SELECTING A NURSE

When a person is seriously sick or in need of special treatment, such as a surgical operation, he usually goes to a hospital. There nursing care is given by professional registered nurses, with the aid sometimes of student nurses, practical nurses, or nurse's aides. At home, unless the patient is critically ill, a full-time professional registered nurse is not usually employed; instead, a part-time professional nurse or a full-time licensed practical nurse may care for the patient.

Professional Registered Nurses

A registered nurse (sometimes called a trained, graduate, or professional nurse) is licensed by the state to practice after completion of an accredited course of training in a school of nursing connected with a registered hospital and passing a state board examination. The initials "R.N." stand for registered nurse. These nurses may be called for duty in homes through nurses' registries. Part-time or hourly professional regis-

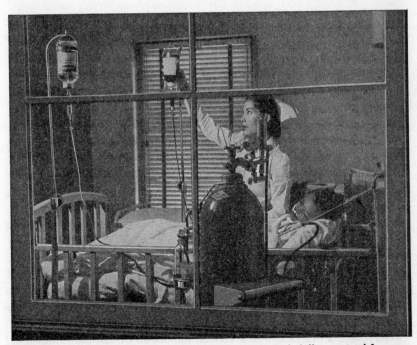

Registered professional nurses are trained in technical skills required for care of the sick.

tered nurses may also be obtained through the professional nurses' registry, a hospital registry, the Visiting Nurse Association, or a doctor.
(Nurses' registries or Visiting Nurse Associations are listed in the telephone directory.)

Public Health or Visiting Nurses

Visiting or public health nurses are professional registered nurses who
will visit the home during the day either to give nursing care, or to teach
someone to give care, or both. Their work in the home is in coöperation
with the family doctor. They will consult with the home nurse regarding
any health problem in the family. They will show how to provide the nursing treatments ordered by the doctor and how to care for a newborn baby
and the mother, a chronically ill patient, or other patient. They will also
supervise the care given by a practical nurse or the home nurse. If the
visiting or public health nursing association is not listed in the telephone
book, call the health department and ask how to obtain a public health
nurse. The charge for public health or visiting nurse service varies in different communities but is usually low and on a cost-per-visit basis. Free
or part-pay service is usually available also to those unable to pay the
full cost.

Practical Nurses

Nurses who have had several months' training in a school of practical
nursing, have passed a state examination, and are licensed to practice
may be obtained for the home nursing of patients who are not critically
ill. However, the supply of these well-prepared practical nurses is limited,
and some states do not license them to practice at all. As a result, many
women calling themselves practical nurses work for hire and sometimes
do not know enough about illness to be safe attendants in the sickroom.
One should be sure one is employing a licensed practical nurse or one that
is recommended by a doctor.

Practical nurses are not expected or prepared to carry out highly skilled
nursing procedures or to be responsible for critically ill patients except as
assistants to registered nurses. They can be of great help, however, in
caring for the moderately ill patient and the chronically ill, and in assisting with the household duties related to the patient's comfort.

To obtain a practical nurse, consult the doctor or call the professional
nurses' registry if there is one, the Visiting Nurse Association, or the local
hospital.

Men Nurses

There are qualified registered men nurses and licensed practical men nurses. Occasionally a male patient prefers care from a man or, in the doctor's opinion, care by a man will be necessary. The same precautions in obtaining service should be taken as when employing a woman. Usually the doctor will recommend the man nurse; there are not as yet many available for private home care.

Home Nurses

Many times a professional or practical nurse is not needed or not available to care for a sick person at home. The responsibility for nursing care then usually falls on the mother of the family, but other members of the household, a relative, or a neighbor may have to help out, especially if it is the mother who is sick.

Whenever there is a sick person in the home, it is beneficial for the patient if other members of the family coöperate in giving help. This is particularly true of young people, who, if they have some understanding of the needs of the sick, can contribute toward the patient's well-being and at the same time gain experience and satisfaction through carrying some of the responsibility.

To avoid confusion and misunderstanding, one person should be designated as the home nurse and should be charged with the major responsibility of the patient's care. Even though she will sometimes require help, she should plan the patient's day, see that the doctor's orders are carried out, keep him informed about the patient's condition, and see that the surroundings of the patient are the best that can be provided.

The home nurse should be calm and careful. She should give proper attention to the patient's welfare and arrange her schedule so that she also can meet other family needs. She should talk with the doctor in private, and learn from him just what the course of the illness is likely to be, what he wants her to do, and where she can reach him quickly if necessary.

The home nurse should be in good health herself. This is essential for her own sake and the safety of the patient. A person in a rundown condition, recovering from an operation, illness, or childbirth, should not attempt home nursing if it can possibly be avoided. Nor should anyone with a cold, sore throat, cough, or heart condition undertake it.

In some cases the doctor will prefer that someone other than the home nurse cook for the family to help prevent the spread of infection. Occasionally, if a member of the household is a food handler in a restaurant or food store, he may be restrained from such employment during quarantine. Health regulations concerning communicable diseases may vary in different communities.

The home nurse should not sleep in the same room as the patient unless he needs constant attention during the night, but she should be within

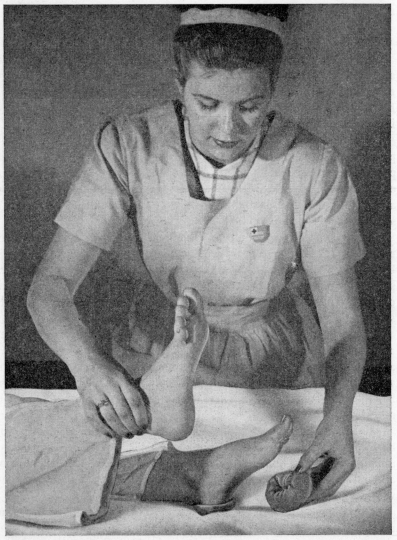

The home nurse should be able to perform simple nursing procedures at home.

call. She should have her own meals regularly and eat properly and should try to sleep 6 hours or more and get outdoors for an hour or so every day. At least once a week she should have complete freedom from her nursing duties for several hours to get away from the home routine. If the patient is a chronic invalid, it is especially important that the home nurse have sufficient time off duty or away from the patient to maintain her own health.

Clothing and Grooming of the Home Nurse

Probably the most important thing for the home nurse to keep in mind when dressing to care for a sick person is her own protection and that of others in the family. Infection, if any is present, must not be passed on to others. Because a sick person may at any time develop a communicable condition that is not always recognized at the start, and because the home nurse is in close contact with the patient and his belongings, her best safeguard is to wear a cover-all washable apron with short sleeves while caring for the patient. This apron or gown should be kept just for this purpose. Any apron, smock, or gown that covers well, is comfortable, has short sleeves, and is washable will serve the purpose. She should wear medium or low-heeled, comfortable shoes with rubber heels so she can walk quietly.

It is not usually necessary for a home nurse to wear a cap, but if her hair is likely to hang down when she is leaning over the patient, she should wear a net or tie her hair back. The home nurse should keep herself and her clothing scrupulously clean and should take precautions against body odors. Other odors such as perfume or tobacco also might be offensive to the patient. Fingernails should be kept reasonably short since long nails may scratch the patient. Rings with settings, bracelets, or a wristwatch should be removed when giving treatments or making beds. If the hands have a tendency to be cold, they should be warmed before the patient is handled. The hands should be kept smooth through the use of cold cream or lotion.

If a mask is necessary for protection, the doctor will advise when and how it should be worn.

Home Nursing Instruction

For nearly 40 years the Red Cross has been teaching people how to carry out simple nursing procedures for the care of the sick at home. The courses do not cover the highly skilled nursing treatments carried out by professional registered nurses, nor do they offer enough instruction to prepare anyone to nurse for hire. For information about these classes, consult the local Red Cross chapter.

MEETING THE EXPENSE OF ILLNESS

Although much illness and many accidents can be prevented by observing good health habits, obtaining early medical attention, and being careful, some illness is to be expected in the life of everyone.

To meet the cost of such emergencies, many persons find it advisable to set aside a certain portion of their regular income each year for medical, dental, and hospital service. This may be done through an insurance plan or savings program.

If medical expenses that arise cannot be met discuss the situation frankly with the doctor, explain the financial circumstances, and tell him how much can be paid on the account each week or month. A similar procedure should be followed in budgeting expenses in connection with specialists and hospitalization.

Information regarding local medical care and hospitalization plans can be obtained from the local medical society, hospital, or Visiting Nurse Association.

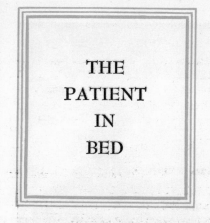

THE PATIENT IN BED

3

ONE of the first aid measures that may well be taken when first observing signs of illness is to put the patient to bed. In bed he will feel more comfortable; he will be warm, quiet, and relaxed, giving the body a chance to rest, build resistance, and help repair any damage. During the first few days in bed, sick people nearly always sleep more than usual, which is highly beneficial since sleep is a great healer. Complications or prolonged illness are often avoided by going to bed promptly when sickness occurs.

Perhaps the most important reason for urging anyone showing signs of illness to go to bed is to prevent the spread of a communicable disease. The early symptoms of many communicable diseases—fever, headache, nausea, sore throat, or running nose—may be the same as those for a cold, an upset stomach, or some other common ailment. To be on the safe side, therefore, the patient should be in a room by himself, if possible, until he feels better or until the doctor gives his diagnosis and orders for care. When the doctor tells a person to stay in bed, he is prescribing a form of treatment that is often as important as medicine, and without which sometimes his medicine can do little good. Sick children should always be put to bed and kept there if possible until the doctor gives his permission for them to get up.

Finally, it is easier for the home nurse to care for a patient who is in bed than to have to look after him as he wanders around the house.

SAVING THE STRENGTH OF THE HOME NURSE

Learning to make the best use of time, material, and money, as well as energy, will aid the home nurse to care for the sick at home as economically and efficiently as possible. (For suggestions on conserving the home nurse's energy, *see* p. 30.) Maintaining good posture at all times helps the body to function without unnecessary strain, thus saving the energy of the home nurse who, in all probability, also may have to carry responsibility for household work.

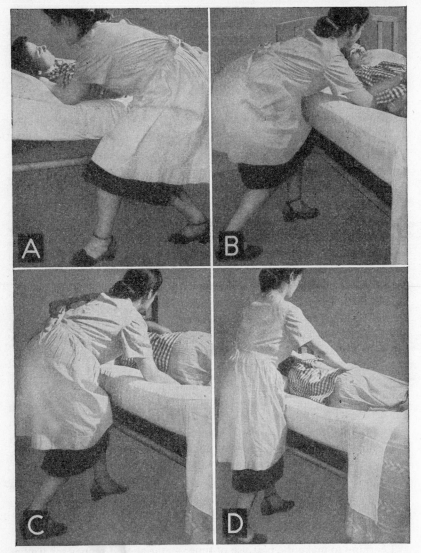

Good posture saves energy of the home nurse.

(A) Helping patient to a sitting position.

(B) Moving patient to near side of bed.

(C) Rolling patient on side.

(D) Rolling patient on back.

BODY POSTURE

Body posture means the position of the parts of the body, head, trunk, arms, and legs, and their relation to one another. Correct posture requires that in standing, sitting, or lying down the natural curves of the spine be maintained, the head be poised comfortably, and the arms and legs be in good alignment with the body.

Body Posture of the Home Nurse.[1] The home nurse should maintain good body posture at all times in performing daily household tasks as well

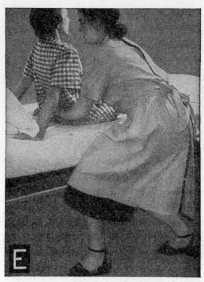

(E) Moving patient toward foot or
head of bed.

as when caring for the patient. Some important points to remember in maintaining good posture are:

1. Keep the chest up and forward to allow ample breathing space. Keep the head comfortably poised.

2. Take the proper stance by standing with the feet separated—toes pointing ahead—one foot forward for balance, when preparing to move a patient.

3. Prepare the muscles for action by taking the proper stance and tensing the abdominal muscles before moving or turning a patient.

4. Bend the knees, keep the back straight, and use the large leg and

[1] Adapted from *Posture and Nursing* by Jessie L. Stevenson, R.N., P.T., New York, Joint Orthopedic Nursing Advisory Service, 1948.

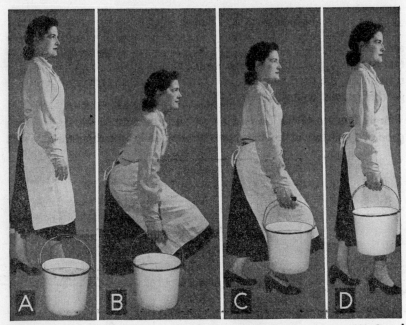

Good posture is important when lifting and carrying objects. (A) Stand close to object. (B) Bend at knees. (C) Lift with back straight. (D) Carry with back straight.

thigh muscles rather than the back muscles to save back strain when moving a patient.

5. Stand close and if possible have the work at about elbow height to save energy.

Body Posture of the Patient.[2] Maintaining good body posture for the bed patient is the responsibility of the home nurse. Some fundamental principles for providing good posture for the patient in bed are:

1. Provide support for the back, shoulders, and head to maintain the natural spinal curves. Keep the chest up and forward to allow ample breathing space. Keep the head comfortably poised.

2. Support the large joints, such as the shoulders, hips, knees, and ankles, to prevent strain.

3. Change the position from time to time to avoid fatigue, prevent continued pressure on any one part of the body, avoid strain on the joints, prevent deformities, provide exercise, and promote circulation.

---

[2] Adapted from *Posture and Nursing* by Jessie L. Stevenson, R.N., P.T., New York, Joint Orthopedic Nursing Advisory Service, 1948.

4. Support the feet at right angles to the legs for comfort and to prevent the tendons from tightening.

5. Encourage the patient to move about in bed if the doctor permits. This will help maintain good joint movement and good muscle tone, and improve the circulation of the blood. The nurse may need to give some passive exercise (exercising of a part of the body, as a muscle or a joint, by another person) to the patient.

Ways of adjusting the body posture of the bed patient so that he will be comfortable and in good alignment are described in Chapter 9, pp. 153–154.

THE SICKROOM

When selecting a room for the patient who is to be in bed for some time, it is well to consider the needs of both the patient and the home nurse and in so far as possible to provide:

1. A sunny, airy room.

2. A room convenient to the bathroom and to the home nurse.

3. Convenient and uncluttered arrangement of personal belongings and furniture, such as the bed, bureau, chairs, bedside table, washstand, washable curtains, and rugs.

4. Quiet.

The patient should be shielded from drafts; glaring surfaces should be avoided and direct lights kept from the patient's eyes. If lights must be shaded, be careful of fire hazards. Rather than using cloth or paper to shade the bulbs, place the lights back of screens on or near the floor.

The sickroom should be kept at a temperature that is comfortable for the patient. It should be aired daily and precautions taken to prevent the patient from chilling. The room temperature should be especially warm when the patient is uncovered for treatments or baths. Gas and oil stoves are not desirable in a sickroom, as they use up oxygen.

Cleanliness and Order

Cleanliness and order are both important to the patient's comfort and welfare. Cleanliness is a safety measure for the patient and other members of the family, while order is not only more pleasant for the patient, but also a timesaving convenience in getting work done. Cleanliness involves keeping the patient and his bed free from perspiration and body discharges, prompt removal of all soiled articles from the room (occasionally the doctor may suggest a deodorant when discharges are offensive), keeping down dust that might carry germs to the patient or from him to other people, and careful washing of the hands both before and after caring for the patient. Even though an illness is not known to be communicable,

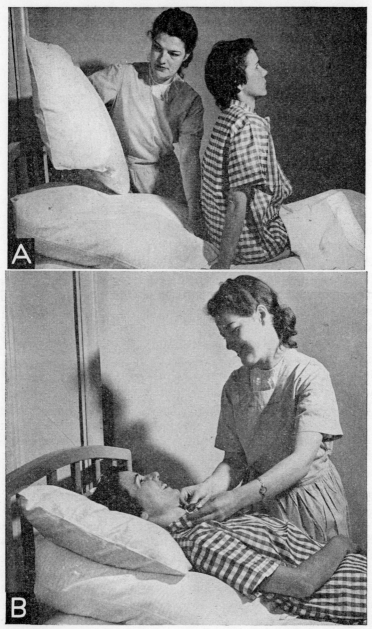

Correct support means more comfort for the patient. (A) Placing pillows for head and shoulder support. (B) Support for shoulders and head makes patient more comfortable.

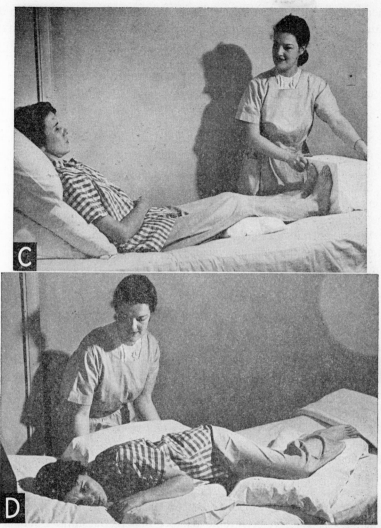

(C) For patient in bed, support is needed for head, back, knees, and feet.
(D) Pillows can be used to support patient lying on side.

there may be disease germs that can be passed on to other people, and precautions must be taken by the generous use of soap and water.

The room should be cleaned in the morning as soon as possible after the patient has been bathed and his bed changed. In cleaning floors and in dusting, care should be taken that the bed is not bumped and that noise is kept to a minimum. The electric vacuum cleaner with its many attachments is ideal for removing dust unless the noise is too disturbing to the patient. If a vacuum cleaner cannot be used, small rugs should be taken from the room to be cleaned. Oiled or damp mops and dustcloths should be used to avoid stirring up the dust. A good dust mop may be made of old stockings or other soft material or an oiled or dampened cloth may be pinned around a broom.

Quiet

Small noises are often more disturbing than loud, accustomed sounds. Particularly disturbing noises are creaking doors, rattling windows, flapping shades, and the click of heels on bare floors.

Sitting on the bed, as well as jarring it, is also disturbing to a sick person, as is whispering or talking just beyond easy earshot. Conversation the patient should not hear should take place completely out of his hearing.

When complete rest in a quiet room is ordered as a part of the treatment, the home nurse should make every effort to see that it is provided for the patient.

THE PATIENT'S BED

The ideal bed for a sick person is one that is high enough to enable the home nurse to give care to the patient without straining her back and neck muscles. If the patient is to be in bed a long time, it is a good idea to get a hospital bed. Often these beds may be purchased or rented from a hospital or supply company. Such a bed has a metal frame, which is easy to clean; it is 36 to 40 inches wide and adjustable so that the patient's head and feet can be raised or lowered mechanically. The legs have casters so that the bed can be easily rolled to a new position.

If a hospital bed is unnecessary or if it is impracticable to obtain one, the home nurse can find a number of ways to elevate a home bed to a height that will enable her to work with ease.

To make the bed higher, cinder blocks, large tin cans partially filled with sand, or specially built wood blocks may be used under each leg when the casters have been removed. (*See* Making Substitute Equipment, p. 202.)

Bedstead and Springs

The standard size single bed is 39 inches wide and 6½ feet long. Longer beds are available for very tall people. A bed that is too short is uncomfortable and leads to bad posture. When necessary, added length may be provided by placing chairs and cushions or other support at the proper height at the foot of the bed if there is no footboard. The springs and mattress must be firm to maintain good body support; a bed that is too soft or one that sags is also uncomfortable and leads to bad posture; the bedpan may sink down or tip under the patient's weight in such a bed. To prevent springs from sagging, a wide board may be placed under the mattress. This board should be the width of the bed and long enough to reach at least from the shoulders to the knees. Wallboard or stiff linoleum may be used for this purpose.

The Mattress

Mattresses may be made of rubber foam or filled with horsehair, felt and cotton, felt and kapok, straw, or corn husks. The two latter fillings grow bumpy with use and need to be renewed frequently. A good mattress pays for itself in comfort and durability.

Good care given to the mattress will prolong its life and help keep it in a sanitary condition. To keep a mattress clean, it should be enclosed in a muslin cover that can be removed and washed. Covers can be bought readymade with zipper closings or can be made at home from a good quality of unbleached muslin and fastened at the end with buttons, snaps, or tape ties. Waterproof coverings are also available.

The mattress should be turned regularly from end to end and from side to side so that pressure and wear will be distributed as evenly as possible. Exposure to the direct air and sunlight once a week will keep it fresh and clean smelling, and the air helps make the filling expand. A thorough brushing with a stiff whisk broom—or better, the use of a vacuum cleaner on the mattress—removes the dust and helps keep the mattress from packing down and growing hard.

If a special mattress is to be purchased for an invalid, the advice of the family doctor or the local hospital may be sought. It pays to buy a good mattress with durable, firm ticking if there is a bedridden invalid in the home. In addition to the mattress cover, a mattress pad of quilted cotton or a washable cotton quilt or blanket should be provided to protect the mattress from moisture or soiling.

Sheets

Sheets of ample size are necessary for both comfort and cleanliness. A safe rule is to have sheets a yard longer and a yard wider than the mattress. A sheet of such dimensions is large enough to tuck under the sides and leave 12 to 18 inches to tuck under the head of the mattress, providing good anchorage for the bottom sheet and sufficient length for the top sheet to fold over and protect the blankets at the head of the bed.

Pillows

The kinds and numbers of pillows will depend upon the patient's needs and desires. A variety of pillows, such as hard, soft, large, and small, may be needed to provide necessary support. They should be kept covered, clean, and fluffed up. When possible, they should be aired in the sun occasionally.

Additional Bed Protection

Whenever a treatment is given in bed or the bedpan is used, or when there is vomiting or other body discharges are present, extra protection will be needed under the patient. This protection may be a sheet of rubber, oilcloth, or pliofilm, a piece of old sheeting or muslin, or several thicknesses of newspaper covered with a large piece of cloth, which can be removed and washed when soiled. Newspapers are not always satisfactory. They afford only limited protection, and the noise of their crackling and tearing may be disturbing to the patient.

Constant protection may be provided by a sheet or strip of oilcloth, rubber, or pliofilm wide enough to reach across the bed and tuck under the mattress and to extend well above and below the area needing protection (usually from the shoulders to the knees). Over this is placed a folded sheet, called a drawsheet, that can be drawn out easily and changed or moved from side to side to present a fresh surface; also, the patient may be moved with the aid of the drawsheet. The rubber sheet and drawsheet should be kept as tight, smooth, and dry as possible to insure the patient's comfort. Sometimes the drawsheet alone is sufficient protection and saves frequent changing of the undersheet; this conserves the energy of both the patient and the home nurse.

Directions for preparing a bed, putting on the drawsheet, and changing the sheets on a bed with a patient in it will be found in Changing the Bed Linen, p. 147.

Blankets

Blankets used in the sickroom should be clean, soft, light in weight, and sufficiently warm for the patient's comfort. Extra covering may be needed for nights or cold weather.

A blanket should be 10 or 12 inches longer and at least 18 inches wider than the bed to allow for ample covering of the body and feet. Since some shrinkage must always be expected, buy the largest blanket available for each bed size. Wool blankets must be washed in warm (never hot), soft water and mild suds. They should be rinsed through clear warm water and then pressed or squeezed to get the water out. Wringing twists the wool fiber and is hard on the blanket. After as much water as possible is squeezed out, the blanket should, whenever possible, be hung outdoors in the fresh air and sunshine to dry.

Cotton blankets are useful in mild weather, but if used in sufficient numbers to be of any value in cold weather they are stiff, heavy, and uncomfortable. They do not absorb moisture as well as wool blankets, and unless the nap is brushed up after they are laundered, they may become rough and irritating to the skin. An extra blanket, which may be flannel or cotton, will be needed for giving treatments to the patient in bed.

Electrically heated blankets, comforters, and foot warmers are now available. If such appliances are used, care should be taken and directions for their use must be followed very carefully and exactly.

Bedspreads

White or colored seersucker or muslin bedspreads are light in weight, easily laundered, and inexpensive, and therefore more suitable for use in illness than a heavy elaborate spread.

THE PATIENT'S PERSONAL NEEDS

The bed patient will need special equipment and clothing to keep him comfortable and contented. Most of this equipment and clothing is available in every home; it is simply a matter of gathering it together and arranging it neatly within the patient's reach or on a tray for the use of the home nurse. The essentials are:

1. Nightgowns, nightshirts, or pajamas. These should be of suitable material that can be washed easily.

2. Bedjacket, sweater, or shawl if the patient is allowed to sit up in bed.

3. A warm bathrobe or dressing gown.

4. Slippers.

5. Toilet articles.

6. Paper tissues and a wastepaper bag for their disposal. (*See* Making a Newspaper Bag, p. 139.)

7. Bell or other call system.

8. Footstool if the bed is high and the patient is allowed in and out of bed.

If the patient is not allowed to go to the toilet or use a commode, a bedpan and a urinal for a boy or man will be needed. (*See* Use of the Bedpan and Urinal for the Bed Patient, p. 162.)

If the patient is not too sick, he should have something to read, writing materials, a radio, and other recreational material. Children may have toys.

The home nurse will find it a great timesaver to assemble on trays the things she needs most frequently; for example, a firm box top will hold the clinical thermometer, a jar of wipes (absorbent cotton, toilet paper, or pieces of clean gauze or rags) or paper tissues, the wastepaper bag, soap, and a jar or pitcher of water. A larger tray can be used for holding the equipment necessary to give a bed bath—towels, washcloth, soap, nail cleaner, rubbing alcohol or body oil, talcum, toothbrush (or other means of cleaning the teeth), dentifrice, brush, and comb. A bedside table is practically a necessity, but a straight chair or an orange crate can be substituted. A bag made like a shoe bag with small and large pockets for articles in constant use can be made and hung within the patient's reach.

If water is not restricted, a covered container of fresh drinking water should always be within reach of the patient.

Often the secret of keeping a bed patient contented is to surround him with the things he needs so that he will not feel dependent on others to supply his needs.

Procedures for the home nurse to follow in caring for a bed patient and instructions on how to give the treatments ordered by the doctor will be found on pp. 135–217.

VISITORS

Visitors may be a great comfort to the patient. However, until the doctor has seen the patient and made a diagnosis, visitors should not be permitted. A person with a communicable disease should not have visitors, for there is not only the danger of exposing the visitor to illness but the risk of the visitor's bringing in a new infection to the already weakened patient. Many doctors forbid maternity patients to have any visitors (except the husband and perhaps close relatives) for the first week after the baby's birth. The home nurse should get the doctor's permission to ask visitors to leave or to bar visitors entirely when she sees the need. Friends will more readily accept the doctor's orders without taking offense. If advisable, the visitor should be instructed before going in to avoid topics of conversation that might be too exciting or depressing to the patient, and it may be necessary to set a time limit on the visit in advance. If this is not done, the nurse should be on the alert for signs of weariness in the patient so that she may tactfully suggest that the visit be ended.

As a rule, visitors should not stay while the patient is eating. It is difficult to carry on a conversation and eat a meal while it is still hot, and also embarrassing to some people to be watched when eating. Visitors should not be present in the sickroom during treatments of any kind unless their help is needed.

The best time for a visit is late in the morning or after the afternoon nap. Visitors should come one at a time and should not stay more than about 20 minutes. The visitor's chair should be placed at a safe distance to avoid direct contact with mouth spray and in such a position that the patient will be able to see his face easily. If the home nurse will speak in moderately low tones, the visitor will usually do likewise. As a rule, it is well to leave the patient alone with his visitor.

Occasionally, well-intentioned friends bring gifts of food and expect the patient to sample it at once. The most tactful thing for the home nurse to say is that she will save the dish for a later meal. But she may wish to prevent a repetition of the gift (which may be food not allowed in the patient's diet) by calling the friend later, thanking her, and suggesting that perhaps the next time her patient would enjoy a particular dish that the doctor has approved.

As a rule, pets should be left out of the sickroom.

CARE OF THE PATIENT IN BED

The Patient's Day

When the care of the sick must be added to household and family duties, establish a schedule that will make it possible to give care to the patient at the time he needs it, adjust the regular duties of the home to avoid conflicts with the patient's care, and utilize the help of other members of the family at the time it is available.

Good planning should include time for the home nurse to get out in the fresh air daily and to have some temporary freedom from responsibilities. She can do her best for the patient when she keeps well and gets sufficient sleep, rest, food, and recreation. Obviously, the routine of the patient's day will vary according to the nature and severity of his illness. But the schedule should cover in general the following things:

1. *Before breakfast care:* Use of the toilet or bedpan, the face and hands washed, the mouth and teeth cleaned, the hair brushed, a glass of water or a hot drink, and the bed straightened.

2. Breakfast.

3. Bath and grooming.

4. Temperature, pulse, and respiration, as ordered by the doctor.

5. Medicines and treatment as ordered.

6. Midmorning nourishment.
7. Rest period.
8. Toilet care.
9. Lunch.
10. Nap or rest period.
11. Midafternoon nourishment.
12. Visitors, if permitted, and in convalescence, some light occupation or diversion.
13. Patient and room put in order before supper.
14. Supper.
15. *Evening and night care* (*see* p. 47).

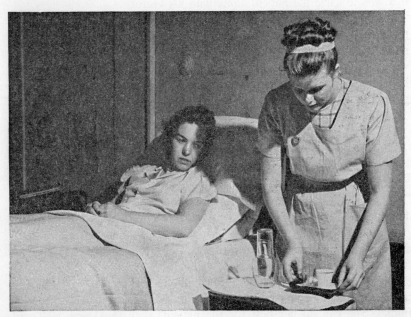

Teenagers can learn to care for the sick at home.

If these main responsibilities are arranged according to some schedule and other household duties fitted around them, the home nurse's time can be used to better advantage and the patient will profit by the regularity and promptness of the service. (The procedures listed above are described in detail in Chapter 9 of this book.)

Preventing Bed Sores

The following precautions should be taken to prevent bed sores:
1. A smooth, clean, dry bed and taut undersheet.

2. A cleansing bath as needed.

3. Back rub and gentle massage of all areas on the body where the skin feels or looks irritated; for example, the base of the spine, the back of the heels, the knees, elbows, shoulders, and occasionally the back of the head or ears in babies and helpless old people. Olive oil or cocoa butter may be used for the massage.

4. Removal of the weight of the bedclothes from the body through use of a pleat for toe space, a foot rest, rolled pillows, or bed cradles. (*See* Making Substitute Equipment: Providing Toe Space for the Bed Patient, p. 208, Providing a Foot Rest, p. 208, *and* Bed Cradle, p. 207.)

5. An air ring or cushion under the base of the spine. This should be slipped into a pillow case and kept dry.

6. A circular pad or "donut" to relieve pressure. (*See* Providing Support and Protection for Pressure Areas, p. 213.)

7. Frequent change of position.

8. Great care in giving and removing the bedpan. The back edge of the bedpan may be padded with a folded towel, the outer edges powdered with talcum powder. The buttocks should be lifted high enough to avoid rubbing against the bedpan.

Care During Hot Weather

A bedridden person may become uncomfortable during hot weather. The home nurse should be aware of this discomfort and provide means of helping the patient to keep as cool as possible. She may use the following measures:

1. Use lightweight, moisture-proof material when bed protection is needed.

2. Use an electric fan with the air stream directed away from the patient.

3. Remove all but lightweight covering.

4. Provide a cotton bed gown.

5. Supply plenty of cool, fresh water and fruit juices if allowed.

6. Give a cool sponge bath (alcohol or water) several times a day if allowed and the time permits.

7. Apply ice to the head in a well-protected bag or other container.

Preparing the Patient for the Night

Everything possible should be done to keep the patient from getting too tired during the latter part of the day, because it may interfere with his rest at night. In general, visitors should be encouraged to come in

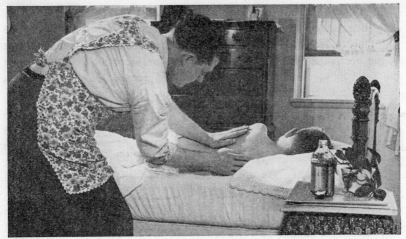

A back rub refreshes and relaxes the patient.

the afternoon rather than in the evening. Light evening nourishment should be given according to the doctor's instructions, after which the patient should be allowed to rest quietly for an hour or so. This may be a good time to put the room in order, remove the flowers and all unnecessary articles, and assemble the material for evening care.

If the patient is able to sleep well and is not seriously ill, it is better to leave him entirely alone at night and to go to him only if he calls. But if he is restless and wakeful or suffering pain, he needs companionship and care. Perhaps a hot water bag at his feet or an extra blanket may be needed. Sometimes a drink of warm milk is especially soothing. A shifting of pillows, a change of position, or a light back rub, using gentle, firm strokes the full length of the spine, may be restful and help to bring on sleep.

A state of mental calmness is as important as physical comfort in preparing the patient for a restful night. The home nurse should keep conversation and activities as restful and relaxing as possible during the latter part of the day and evening. She should assemble the equipment she will need in giving evening care to the patient. Usually this care will include:

1. Taking the temperature if ordered.
2. Giving medicine if ordered.
3. Giving nourishment if permitted.
4. Giving the bedpan.
5. Washing the patient's face and hands and brushing his hair.

6. Helping brush the teeth.

7. Giving a back rub.

8. Changing the nightgown if desired, and putting on a bedjacket if needed.

9. Taking off the spread, putting on an extra blanket and placing a hot water bag to the feet if needed.

10. Arranging the pillows for correct support.

11. If light is needed, arranging it so that it cannot shine on the patient's face, or providing the patient with a means of turning on the light, or giving the patient a flashlight.

12. Seeing that the call bell, fresh drinking water, and reading material (if desired) are handy.

13. Having a bedpan or urinal handy if the patient is able to help himself.

14. Taking flowers out of the room.

15. Putting a silencer on the door.

16. Adjusting the windows so that the air is fresh but not cold and does not blow directly on the patient.

17. Being sure the room is in order, and asking if the patient is comfortable.

18. Recording on the daily record the care given and comments on the patient's day and general condition.

DAILY RECORD FOR THE DOCTOR

The home nurse will be expected by the doctor to keep a daily record of the patient's illness. This record will indicate how the patient feels, behaves, and reacts to treatments during his illness and will include information as to what has been done for him, when it was done, and what was observed about him. The doctor should write his orders for the patient on this record. If he gives them by telephone, the home nurse writes them on the record and the doctor signs his name at his next visit. The home nurse then indicates when she carried out these orders and the results. The home nurse must not trust to memory. She must provide for the doctor an accurate statement of care given and of the patient's reaction. As a patient's condition changes from day to day, this information may have great significance to the doctor in diagnosing a condition and helping the patient get well.

When more than one person is giving care to the patient, this record is absolutely necessary to avoid confusion and misunderstanding in carrying out the orders for the patient, and it is a protection to both patient and nurse. It is well to keep the daily record out of sight of the patient and out of reach of children at all times.

A form for keeping the daily record is shown here, with typical entries filled in. The report covers in general the symptoms observed, treatments given, services rendered, kind of medicine given (also the time and amount), reactions to treatments, nourishment (including liquids), sleep, rest, bowel movements, and bladder output. The temperature is taken and reported as ordered by the doctor. The patient's reactions and the nurse's impressions of the patient's progress should be noted also. The date and hour should always appear.

While this daily report may seem like just one more duty, it is important to the doctor and patient. A simple entry of a symptom observed by a home nurse has been known to save a life. The report should be clear, brief, neat, and accurate. A notebook may be used if the illness is likely to be of long duration.

Daily Record:						Jane Jones
Date and hour	Temp.	Diet　　Medicines　　Treatment			BM	UR	Remarks
10-17-49 8 a.m.	101.4				✓	Throat red and swollen.
8³⁰a.m.		Small glass of orange juice One cup of coffee with cream Small saucer of oatmeal gruel				Jane swallows with difficulty.
10³⁰a.m.					✓	✓	Soft brown stool
11-11³⁰a.m.		Steam inhalation for one half hour				Nose stopped up.
12 noon		Small bowl strained vegetable soup Glass of milk				Jane coughing a good deal, says it is painful in her chest.
1 p.m.		Medicine No. 547- 1 teaspoonful				
4 p.m.	99.6				✓	
4¹⁵ - 4⁴⁵ p.m.		Steam inhalation for one half hour				Coughing less.
6 p.m.						
10-18-49 8 a.m	99.2					Jane slept most of the night

Do not trust to memory. Keep a simple record of the patient's illness.

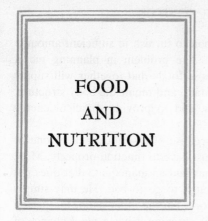

FOOD AND NUTRITION

4

IMPORTANCE OF FOOD

FROM earliest times man has realized that providing food for himself and his family was one of his major tasks. He knew that food sustained life, and he also noticed that a full stomach brought happiness and contentment. He did not, however, understand the relationship of food to his health. It has been the tireless work of the men and women engaged in scientific research who have made man appreciate the body's delicate and efficient mechanism. But it has been largely in the present century that we have gained definite knowledge of nutrition, that is, learned something of the physiological processes by which the body makes food into bone, blood, brain, and brawn.

The human body in its functioning is far more amazing than the finest watch or the most intricate motor. There are, however, similarities between the body and a machine. Our bodies require fuel just as does the motor. Some of us have not stopped to realize that every breath taken, every beat of the heart, every movement of the body requires energy or fuel. Food supplies fuel to yield this energy. The remarkable difference in the human body and the machine is the way in which the body can repair its own worn parts. The motor, when it needs a new part or when an old part requires repair, must remain idle until the damaged part is repaired or replaced by the mechanic. The human body, however, is able to repair itself to a large degree.

Whether well or ill, the body must have certain specific substances to carry on its various functions, including the provision of fuel and materials for growth and repair of itself. The sources of these substances, called nutrients, are food and water. The choice of food, therefore, should be made first of all to meet these needs. This does not mean that preference, custom, convenience, availability, and cost must be set aside and the diet limited to a few foods. On the contrary, if the food needs of the body as well as the composition of the different commonly used foods are understood, the selection of an adequate diet leads to the use of a greater variety of foods.

51

No single food can be depended upon to furnish in sufficient amounts all the nutrients required for health. The problem in planning meals for the day, therefore, is to choose those foods that together will supply all the nutrients needed to build, maintain, and repair the body structure, to regulate the many body processes, and to provide sufficient energy for the activities of the body.

Sometimes the body becomes ill because of a serious lack of one or more of these specific substances it must have to function properly. More often the person who for some time has had an inadequate diet does not become critically ill or even sick enough to go to bed. He may simply feel run down, tired, and unable to work. On the other hand, the person who is selecting his food wisely and is enjoying it has a good chance of feeling and keeping well. A scientist in the field of nutrition has said, "No one in his right mind will deliberately continue to eat foods that he knows will damage his heart, nerves, arteries, stomach, brain, and other vital organs, but he may do so in case of ignorance or doubt. It would be folly, therefore, to condone letting civilized people go on eating whatever foods merely appeal to an immediate sense of pleasure. Even the simplest appraisal of food in terms of enjoyment and cost cannot be divorced, in fact, from effects upon health. Every intelligent layman is entitled to know these basic relationships, despite the fact that new discoveries are extending man's horizons in this area almost daily."[1]

USEFUL INFORMATION

This chapter discusses food and nutrition for the entire family as well as for the patient. The basic information given here should be useful not only to a home nurse but to others interested in planning good meals. Simple guides to the selection of proper food for the family as well as for the patient are given. Tables list the foods allowed in the standard diets most often ordered by doctors and suggest meals using these foods.

Meals for the family as well as for the ill and convalescent are worthy of the homemaker's time and thought, not only because delicious meals are popular but also because food is important to the health of her family. As a home nurse she has in her hands one of the important secrets for helping the patient to recover and keep well.

GOOD COOKING

Every woman who keeps house should own a reliable cookbook. When she makes a new dish or is learning to cook, she should try to follow

[1] From an address given at Columbia University, 1949, by Dr. C. G. King, Scientific Director, The Nutrition Foundation, Inc., New York.

very carefully the directions given in the cookbook. After she becomes experienced and skilled at cooking, she can afford to take "a pinch of this" and "about so much of that." But until her eye is trained, she may ruin much good food by careless mixing and improper methods of cookery.

CHOOSING FOOD FOR HEALTH

How can a person know when she is choosing the right food to keep herself and her family in good health? The planning of meals that will include the right combination of foods is not a difficult task. It can be simple when a general pattern is developed and followed.

For convenience, foods that are alike may be grouped together. Many reading this book will have heard of the basic food groups or have seen

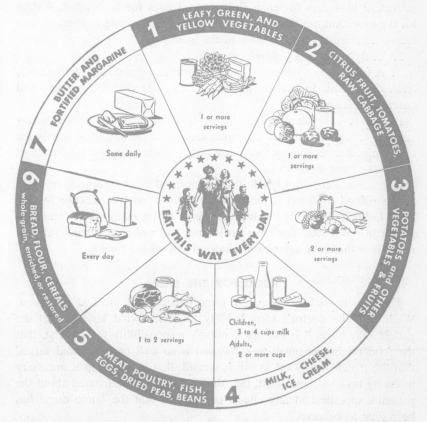

The basic seven food groups. (From National Food Guide, Issued by Bureau of Human Nutrition and Home Economics, U. S. Department of Agriculture.)

a basic seven food chart.[2] Foods found in each of these essential food groups may be used interchangeably, thus allowing many choices within each group. The homemaker can easily become familiar with the chart, The Basic Seven Food Groups, shown here. She will find it helpful to check the day's food with the chart in order to see that some food from each group has been included in the meals served her family.

Three of the food groups in the chart mentioned above should be especially checked by every person responsible for providing meals, because studies of the buying and eating habits of American families have shown that these are the ones most often neglected. The three food groups that may need particular emphasis in many families are:

1. Milk to drink and to eat in prepared dishes. Meals each day should provide 3 to 4 cups for each child, 2 to 3 cups for each adult, 4 cups for the expectant mother, and 5 to 6 cups for the nursing mother. (A cup means a measuring cup or an 8 ounce glass.)

2. Leafy green and yellow vegetables.

3. A food rich in vitamin C, such as oranges, grapefruit, or tomatoes, fresh or canned. In season, pears, peaches, strawberries, melons, and other fresh fruits.

Fish liver oils like cod-liver oil or the vitamin-D concentrates (increased strength in reduced amounts) are also important, particularly for children and expectant mothers. The family doctor can best advise about the amount and kinds to use.

The use of *iodized salt* (salt in which natural iodine has been replaced in the refined product) is recommended. Look on the package for the word *iodized*. The body needs a tiny bit of iodine every day. Vegetables grown in some localities have no iodine, and ordinary refined salt has none. It is therefore safer to use iodized salt all the time.

FOOD FOR THE SICK

Feeding the sick is always an important part of medical treatment. While it is the doctor's responsibility to decide what kind of diet the patient may have, it is the home nurse's responsibility to see, first, that the food retains its nutritive value and is so well prepared and served that the patient will want to eat it; second, that he has help if necessary in taking his food; and third, that the doctor is kept informed about the patient's appetite and any effects of the diet that the home nurse has been able to observe.

[2] A free copy of the leaflet, *National Food Guide,* AIS 53, may be obtained from the Office of Information, U. S. Department of Agriculture, Washington 25, D. C.

The doctor should always be asked, if he does not remember to tell the home nurse, what kind of diet the patient may have. In some cases he will simply say, "A regular diet; give him any thing he wants to eat." Or he may direct that the patient be given his usual meals in small servings. He will mean, of course, that the patient may be offered food at regular hours, and that his favorite foods may be included. The home nurse will most likely be able to give him tempting amounts of many of the same foods included in the meals for the family. It is important that the patient enjoy his meals, but it is equally necessary that he be properly nourished. If he is well enough, the patient may be interested in having someone explain what foods will help him get well and why some foods are more important than others.

Planning meals for a sick person or one who is convalescing is a necessary, though not always easy, task. It may help if the home nurse can imagine herself in the patient's place. She will then recall, for example, how the appetite is affected by lack of exercise and illness.

• Serving Meals to the Patient

When one is weak and hungry, waiting for food is extremely trying. If the stomach is entirely empty, its walls touch, causing pangs of hunger. To reduce such distress and to aid the home nurse, the patient's food schedule should be set up apart from the family mealtime. When he is able to take a light or full diet, he may often be served some of the same food the family is to have. If he is not able to go to the table, his tray should be prepared and served before the family meal and while the food is hot and most palatable. High seasoning and rich sauces should be omitted. Be sure the food served him is seasoned simply, looks attractive, and tastes good.

The appearance of the tray may affect the appetite favorably or unfavorably. Dishes should be attractive and related to the size of the tray. The tray cloth and napkin should be spotless. Paper tray cloths and napkins are convenient and inexpensive. If several different kinds of decorated napkins are used alternately, they will provide an element of interest and color that is pleasing to adults as well as children. The habit of placing a fresh flower, an interesting newspaper clipping, or a little favor on the tray may help to make mealtime an occasion to which the patient looks forward with pleasure.

Since the sight, aroma, and taste of food that the patient enjoys aid his digestion, the home nurse should try to serve foods the patient likes, if the diet allows them. Select fresh, colorful foods. Cook vegetables in a

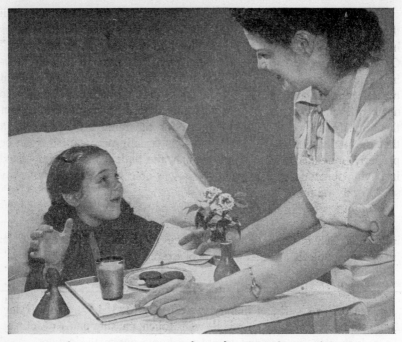

An attractive tray stimulates the patient's appetite.

small amount of water and just before serving. See to it that each food is as appetizing as possible, make the tray attractive, and provide a pleasant atmosphere for the meal.

Before the tray is brought to the patient, he should be allowed to use the bedpan, if desired. After this, his hands and face should be washed so that he will feel relaxed and refreshed for his meal. Then the room and bed should be put in order, the back rest or pillows adjusted to his comfort, and the bed table arranged conveniently. The patient will have less difficulty in digesting his food when he is calm and relaxed.

The average person prefers to feed himself, but helpless and weak patients or small children must be assisted. The tray should be placed where the patient can see his food, and the food should be given to him in small bites, alternating various foods as he would do if feeding himself. Unless he is weak, he may prefer to hold his bread and butter and eat it when he wishes. Usually he will wish to wipe his own mouth.

If the patient is too ill to be propped up in a sitting position with pillows, the nurse may place her hand under the pillow, raise the head slightly, and hold the glass or spoon to the lips. The patient's head should be allowed to drop back into a comfortable position. The neck must not be bent forward since this interferes with swallowing. Liquids served hot must be only pleasantly hot, not so hot that they will burn the lips and tongue. If the head cannot be raised, or if the patient prefers it, a drinking tube may be used. Glass drinking tubes or soda straws may be bought at the drug store. Care should be used when feeding a small child or a patient who is delirious, as he may bite the tube. A small teapot or cream pitcher makes a convenient drinking cup for the bed patient. Turning the head to one side may help the patient swallow, if he is being fed from a drinking tube.

The kind and amount of food eaten should always be written on the patient's record so that the doctor may determine whether the patient is taking enough nourishing food.

A patient who has an injury or illness that merely keeps him from exercising and has no effect on his appetite is likely to eat more than he needs. As a result, he may put on too much weight and also may be troubled with constipation. To correct this condition, the doctor may order foods for the patient that have a high roughage content to aid elimination and may greatly increase the amount of liquids, especially fruit juices. He may also ask that the more concentrated foods, such as fats and sweets, be given sparingly so that the patient will not gain too much weight.

The Doctor's Diet Orders

It is best to ask the doctor to write down all his orders, including the kind of diet the patient may have. The home nurse has many duties and should not depend on her memory in carrying out the doctor's orders. Often the doctor prescribes a liquid, soft, light, or full diet. The home nurse should be sure that she understands what foods are to be included in such diets. Since food is an important part of the treatment in many illnesses, the doctor's directions as to diet should be followed with as much care as those given for medication.

When the doctor orders a special diet, the home nurse may want someone to help her plan meals that not only meet the patient's needs but fit the family's food habits and budget. The home nurse may be able to obtain help from the nutritionist on the staff of the local Red Cross chapter, the local health department, or some other community agency. The dietitian at the hospital will usually be glad to make suggestions for carrying out the doctor's diet orders, especially when the patient is about to return to his home from the hospital.

Table 1*—STANDARD DIETS USUALLY ORDERED BY DOCTORS

Type of Food	Full Diet	Light Diet	Soft Diet	Full Liquid Diet
Fruits	All	All cooked and canned fruits, citrus fruits, bananas	Fruit juices; cooked and canned fruits (without seeds, coarse skins, or fiber); bananas	Fruit juices, strained
Cereals and cereal products	All	Cereals, dry or well cooked; spaghetti and macaroni, not highly seasoned	Same as Light Diet	Gruels, strained
Breads	All	Enriched and whole-wheat bread, soda crackers	Same as Light Diet	
Soups and broths	All	All	Broth, strained cream soups	Same as Soft Diet
Meat, fish, and poultry	All	Tender steaks and chops, lamb, veal, ground or tender beef, bacon, chicken, sweetbreads, liver, fish	Tender chicken, fish, and sweetbreads; ground beef and lamb	
Eggs	Eggs cooked in all ways	Soft-cooked eggs	Same as Light Diet	Eggnogs
Dairy products	Milk, sweet and acid; cream; butter; cheese of all kinds	Milk, sweet and acid; cream; butter; cottage and cream cheese; Cheddar cheese used in cooking	Same as Light Diet	Milk, sweet and acid; cream
Vegetables	All, including salads	Cooked vegetables: asparagus, peas, string beans, spinach, carrots, beets, squash Salads: tomato and lettuce Potatoes: boiled, mashed, creamed, scalloped, baked	Cooked vegetables: same as Light Diet Salads: none Potatoes: same as Light Diet	
Desserts	All	Ices, ice cream, junket, cereal puddings, custard and gelatin, simple cakes, plain cookies	Same as Light Diet	Ices, ice cream, gelatin, junket, and custard
Beverages	All	Tea, coffee, and cocoa; coffee substitutes; milk and milk beverages; carbonated beverages	Same as Light Diet	Same as Light Diet

58

* The data in Table 1 are from the table, Foods Allowed in Standard Hospital Diets in *Nutrition in Health and Disease*, 11th ed., 1950, and are included through the courtesy of the authors: Lenna F. Cooper, Edith M. Barber, and Helen S. Mitchell, and the publishers, J. B. Lippincott Co., Philadelphia.

Table 2* — Typical Menus for Diets Usually Ordered by Doctors

Full Diet	Light Diet	Soft Diet	Full Liquid Diet
Breakfast	*Breakfast*	*Breakfast*	*Breakfast*
Fresh pear	Orange	Orange juice	Strained orange juice
Oatmeal with milk or cream	Oatmeal with milk or cream	Oatmeal with milk or cream	Strained oatmeal gruel with milk or cream
Scrambled eggs	Soft scrambled eggs	Soft scrambled eggs	Coffee with cream and sugar
Buttered whole-wheat toast	Buttered whole-wheat toast	Buttered whole-wheat toast	
Coffee with cream and sugar	Coffee with cream and sugar	Coffee with cream and sugar	
			10 A.M.
Dinner	*Dinner*	*Dinner*	Eggnog
Vegetable soup	Vegetable soup	Strained vegetable soup	*Dinner*
Roast veal	Roast veal	Ground beef	Broth with rice
Mashed potato	Mashed potato	Mashed potato	Ginger ale with ice cream
Buttered broccoli	Buttered carrots	Buttered carrots	Coffee with cream and sugar
Tomato salad with French dressing	Tomato salad with French dressing	Whole-wheat or white bread	
Whole-wheat, rye, or white bread	Whole-wheat, rye, or white bread	Butter	
Butter	Butter	Vanilla ice cream with chocolate sauce	
Peppermint stick ice cream	Peppermint stick ice cream	Milk	*3 P.M.*
Milk	Milk		Malted milk or buttermilk
Supper	*Supper*	*Supper*	*Supper*
Cream of pea soup with crackers	Cream of pea soup with crackers	Cream of pea soup with crackers	Strained cream of pea soup
Macaroni au gratin	Macaroni au gratin	Macaroni au gratin	Plain gelatin with whipped cream
Head lettuce salad with Russian dressing	Head lettuce salad with French dressing	Buttered beets	Tea with cream and sugar
Bread	Bread	Bread	
Butter	Butter	Butter	
Fruit gelatin	Fruit gelatin	Plain gelatin with whipped cream	
Tea with cream and sugar	Tea with cream and sugar	Tea with cream and sugar	*10 P.M.*
			Hot cocoa

59

* The data in Table 2 are from the table, Typical Menus for Standard Hospital Diets in *Nutrition in Health and Disease*, 11th ed., 1950, and are included through the courtesy of the authors: Lenna F. Cooper, Edith M. Barber, and Helen S. Mitchell, and the publishers, J. B. Lippincott Co., Philadelphia.

The tables provided here should be helpful to the home nurse. Table 1 lists the foods usually allowed on the standard diets known as liquid, soft, light, and full. Table 2 suggests meals that follow these diets.

Food When the Patient Has a Fever

When the body temperature rises above the level accepted as "normal," we say a person has a fever. The old saying, "starve a fever," is out of date. Although care must be taken during the fever stage of illness to include only foods that can be easily digested, usually enough food can be given to the patient to bring him through reasonably well nourished, not thin and gaunt as was often the case with a patient in our grand-mother's day.

To put as little strain on digestion as possible and to increase the fluid intake, a liquid diet given at two-hour intervals is often prescribed for the patient with a fever. (See Tables 1 and 2, pp. 58–59.) Fruit juices, moderately strong tea or coffee with cream and sugar, carbonated drinks, strained soups, milk, and ice cream may be included. The doctor may ask that sugar be added to the milk. A gruel made by cooking cereal thoroughly, straining, and adding water or milk to make it quite thin is popular in a liquid diet. Patients often dislike or tire of sweet foods, and the blandness of gruels is a welcome change. As the patient progresses toward recovery, the doctor may allow buttered toast, breakfast cereals without bran, soft-cooked eggs, strained vegetables, and baked or mashed potatoes, thoroughly cooked. The meals gradually change from the liquid or soft diet pattern to the light and eventually the full or general diet. The doctor will order, as early in the illness as he considers wise, a diet that is high in protein and caloric value. He does so because during fever some body protein is destroyed, and the need for body fuel is increased above normal.

Feeding a Sick Child

A sick child may be fussy about his food, so it seems sensible not to be too insistent about his eating and to offer him at first only small amounts of the simple foods suggested by the doctor. A child not acutely ill will appreciate food served in unusual ways and on different china with colorful paper napkins and covers.

It may be necessary to serve refreshments between meals to be sure the patient is getting enough nourishment and the right variety of foods. The doctor will prescribe the diet, just as he does the medicine, for a sick baby or child. The sick child's diet usually includes fruit juices, skim or whole milk, milk toast, soft-cooked eggs, cereals strained and thinned to a gruel, custards, gelatin desserts, junket, and ice cream.

The doctor may suggest that a child who is troubled with vomiting be offered small amounts of liquids, in sips. If he asks for solid food, he may be started on a small cracker or thin gruel. For the child with whooping cough, the doctor will frequently order the home nurse to give nourishing food immediately after vomiting so he may have an opportunity to benefit from it before his next attack of coughing and vomiting. Solid foods are often retained more easily than liquids by the child with whooping cough.

When a child is recovering from an illness, one of the first signs is a returning appetite; he may suddenly demand food and more food. Meals should, however, be small at first and the amount increased slowly, since the digestive system cannot suddenly handle an overload. Small between-meal feedings should be provided, and the child gradually returned to a full diet.

FOOD FOR THE EXPECTANT MOTHER

The home nurse, whether caring for herself or for others, should know that the expectant mother who chooses her food wisely is not only more likely to remain in fine health but has a better chance of giving birth to a normal, healthy baby. Reliable studies have shown that the diet of the expectant mother affects the physical condition of the baby. A person who is well nourished before pregnancy, eats an adequate diet during this period, and has a cheerful outlook on life may not have the nausea or the early-morning sickness often associated with pregnancy. It is particularly important that the diet supply enough of the two nutrients, calcium and protein. Milk is the richest source of calcium and also contains the highest quality protein. Dry skim milk and evaporated milk, used generously, will add calcium and protein of low cost and high value to the diet. The expectant mother should also eat the foods that are rich in iron, such as eggs, liver and other meats, green leafy vegetables, dark molasses, and the whole-grain breads and cereals.

The diet recommended for the expectant mother is of special importance because it supplies generous amounts of protein, minerals, and vitamins to build new body structure for the mother and baby. Protein is particularly important since the mother accumulates a reserve which is evidently a safety factor in preparation for delivery, for the period after birth, and for successful lactation (nursing her baby). It is therefore essential that the expectant mother eat the foods rich in protein, minerals, and vitamins.

She requires a quart of milk a day, or double the amount needed by another adult. Fruits, vegetables, whole-grain breads and cereals, meat and fish, eggs, milk, and cheese provide the protein, minerals, and vitamins to furnish these building materials for the unborn child and for the expectant mother herself. If the mother does not have all these foods in her diet or has them in insufficient amounts, both she and the baby suffer from the lack. Authorities generally agree that when the mother's diet is inadequate, the baby draws its building material from the tissues of the mother's body. It is important that the expectant mother's diet be fully adequate.

It is true that the expectant mother usually gains weight, and the amount and kinds of food she eats largely determine whether her gain is excessive. Her caloric requirements are only about 20 per cent or 1/5 above her usual needs. To keep her weight where the doctor wants it and at the same time maintain good health, her meals should be planned around the three food groups listed on p. 54, plus just enough of other foods to keep that weight. If she is gaining weight too fast, she will do well to eat less, particularly of fats, starches, and sweets. The expectant mother or the home nurse may wish to get a copy of the booklet, *Prenatal Care,* Children's Bureau, Publication No. 4, from the Superintendent of Documents, Government Printing Office, Washington 25, D. C.

In addition to the foods listed here, many doctors now prescribe some form of vitamin D in the diet of the expectant mother. This may be a tasteless concentrate or a capsule containing cod or other fish-liver oil. Sometimes calcium pills are ordered by the physician. It should be remembered that these calcium preparations only supplement the diet and are not a substitute for the milk. It takes some 25 to 30 of the usual calcium pills to supply the amount of calcium in 1 quart of milk. The doctor may also ask that the mother take an iron "tonic" or capsules high in iron content, or suggest foods rich in iron.

It is now known that the growing fetus (unborn baby) stores iron during the last 2 months of pregnancy, probably in his liver. He stores enough, in fact, to last him 5 or 6 months after birth. The doctor may decide that the expectant mother needs additional iron so that her body will not be drained of this important mineral in order to supply the baby with all he needs to store up a reserve. Good food sources of iron are liver, kidney, heart (serve one of these at least once a week), other meats, eggs, dried apricots, raisins, molasses, leafy and green vegetables, dried beans, peas, lentils, and potatoes.

Milk is an extremely valuable food in the diet. There are many ways to take the daily quart in addition to drinking it. Whether fresh pasteurized, dried, or evaporated milk is chosen, it is well worth whatever it may cost. Skim milk may be used if the diet includes butter or fortified margarine to replace the fat and vitamin A lacking in both dry and liquid skim milk. In many foods prepared with milk only a relatively small amount is used. Many expectant mothers like to drink two or three glasses a day and then use the remainder of the four cups of milk in cooking. A generous 1 inch cube of cheese such as American Cheddar yields approximately the same amount of body-building material as a cup of milk. A whole-grain or enriched cereal may be cooked in milk instead of water; this adds to the flavor and food value of the cereal. Desserts made with milk, such as sherbets, ice cream, custards, or rice pudding, may also be served, unless the person is trying to cut down on sweets.

The milk used will add to the intake of fluids. Because the body of the expectant mother must eliminate the baby's waste products as well as her own, liquids are an absolute "must." Part of this requirement for liquid can be in the form of milk, tea, coffee, and fruit juices. Each glass of liquid, including water, should be counted when reporting to the doctor the amount of liquid taken daily. Water usually may be taken as freely as desired; however, the doctor may give the expectant mother special directions about water.

The diet recommendations outlined above are made for the average expectant mother. Any changes made by the doctor who knows the special needs of the patient should be carefully noted and followed.

FOOD FOR THE NURSING MOTHER

The home nurse should realize that breast-feeding is especially satisfying for a mother because she knows that she is supplying life-giving nourishment to her baby. The amount of breast milk is usually increased when the food eaten by the mother is adequate.

Well-planned family meals can take care of the dietary requirements of the nursing mother. She needs to drink more than the usual amount of liquid every day, to use more milk (about 1½ quarts to drink and in cooked foods), and to eat additional protein foods such as meat, seafood, poultry, eggs, milk, and cheese. If the foods listed on p. 54 are generously represented in her meals, and she eats enough protein and the right amount of other foods to keep a desirable body weight, she will meet her own needs and usually will have plenty of milk for her baby—provided she really wants to nurse him and has no medical or social reasons for not nursing him.

Her appetite will usually be excellent, and, as a rule, she can eat all she wants. However, if she finds that she is gaining weight, she should cut down on sweets and fats until her weight remains constant. Many women *lose* weight while nursing a baby. If the doctor does not want her to lose weight, she should eat more food and probably should rearrange her schedule so that she may lie down for a short period once or twice a day.

Sample Menu for the Nursing Mother

Breakfast: Whole orange or juice, or half a grapefruit; cooked or dry cereal with top milk; one or two eggs (seven weekly); enriched or whole-wheat bread with a spread; glass of milk; coffee or tea.

Midmorning: Glass of tomato or fruit juice.

Luncheon or supper: Thick soup; sandwich (cheese, meat, or peanut butter); cooked or fresh fruit; milk, cocoa, or milk and coffee mixed drink.

Midafternoon: Some fruit or a beverage such as milk, ginger ale, or hot or iced tea.

Dinner: Generous serving of main protein dish (meat, seafood, poultry, eggs, or cheese—use cooked, dried beans, peas, or lentils once a week, if desired); leafy green or yellow vegetable; potatoes; salad of mixed greens, cole slaw, or tomatoes and cucumbers; fresh or cooked fruit and cheese, or other desserts; milk; and tea or coffee.

Bedtime: Milk, cold or warm, as desired.

FEEDING THE CONVALESCENT

It is sometimes hard to find just the foods that a convalescent will enjoy; yet nourishing food is imperative in the repair of the body. The home nurse can try serving small amounts of one or two favorite foods. If the convalescent is able to sit at the family table for one meal, the sociability may improve his appetite. The home nurse should see that his diet includes the essential foods, such as milk, fruit, vegetables, and a protein food. Midmorning and midafternoon refreshments can be tried, unless this spoils his appetite for his regular meals. The home nurse should cater to the patient's special likes in food as far as she can, if the diet ordered by the doctor allows.

Frequently, a high-nourishment or high-caloric diet is ordered following illness. If there has been great prostration (complete exhaustion), weakness, and loss of weight, the doctor may suggest especially nourishing foods. Such a diet, however, does not call for rich foods. The weakened digestive system is easily upset by too much food or by foods very rich in fat and sugar. It is better to add between-meal feedings than to attempt to stuff the patient.

Sample Menu for a High-nourishment Diet

On waking or at breakfast: Fruit juice or whole fruit.

Breakfast: Hot cereal such as oatmeal or whole-wheat cereal, with top milk or cream; egg, if desired; buttered toast and jam or jelly; coffee or tea with cream and sugar.

Midmorning: Tomato or fruit juice and crackers spread with peanut butter, cheese, or jam.

Dinner: Cream soup, such as corn, tomato, or chicken; tender meat (lamb, beef, or veal), fish or other seafood, poultry, or a cheese dish; a baked potato with butter; any leafy, green or yellow vegetable; a baked apple or apple pudding, or plain or stewed fruit; enriched or whole-wheat bread with butter, as desired.

Midafternoon: Thin bread and butter sandwich; cocoa, tea, or a fruit drink.

Supper: Poached egg on toast, if an egg was omitted at breakfast, or plain egg soufflé; bread and butter or milk toast; a small salad of any kind; milk, flavored or plain; ice cream, custard, or cooked fruit.

Before sleep: Warm milk and a buttered cracker or bread.

FEEDING THE AGING AND CHRONICALLY ILL

Food for those who get little exercise should be served at regular intervals and prepared rather simply. Many elderly people prefer to eat their main meal at noon.

It is important that the older person's diet be fully adequate, that is, supplies his body with all the essential food substances. Checking his diet occasionally for the basic foods and especially the three food groups listed on p. 54 will help insure adequacy. His meals can usually be chosen from the food prepared for the family, unless the physician has ordered a special diet. High seasoning can be omitted from his meats, and heavier desserts replaced by fresh or stewed fruit. Food is often one of the principal pleasures left to the older person, and he should as nearly as possible be given his accustomed foods. However, he should be encouraged to cut down on quantities and on rich foods and heavy sweets to keep his weight near or below the average for his height at his age. The doctor who knows the older person can best advise on the proper weight for him. If cheese, fish, and eggs as well as milk are in the diet, meat or poultry may be reduced to two or three servings a week. Tender, finely chopped meat, liver, and fowl are relished by some because they are easy to chew.

It is especially important that the bedridden patient be kept on a well-balanced but nonfattening diet or he may grow heavy and more helpless. Special diets for certain conditions such as constipation or high blood pressure may be ordered by the doctor.

Provide diversions and occupations for this group of patients so that food and the description of symptoms do not become an absorbing interest leading either to overweight, finicky food habits, or enjoyment of invalidism.

DIET IN SPECIAL ILLNESSES

Such diseases as diabetes and kidney ailments require special diets that are a major part of the medical treatment. The doctor will prescribe such diets in detail, and other foods should not be given to the patient. It will often be easier for the person on a restricted diet if only the foods he can eat are served in his presence.

The doctor may, for example, order a high-protein diet, particularly for some kidney diseases. Such foods as meat, fish and other seafoods, poultry, eggs, cheese, and milk will be emphasized in the high-protein diet. The home nurse should, of course, provide this diet carefully if the doctor orders it. She should check with him often to find how long he wishes the diet continued.

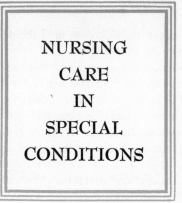

NURSING
CARE
IN
SPECIAL
CONDITIONS

5

THE PATIENT WITH A COM-MUNICABLE DISEASE

THE nursing care of a patient with a communicable disease differs little from that given any other sick person if the home nurse is following all the preventive measures recommended in the nursing procedures described in this book. The main difference is that after the diagnosis has been made, she is *sure* of danger of infection. The length and type of illness will largely determine what special protective measures to take. In general, communicable diseases may be spread through discharges either from the nose and throat or from the bowel and bladder. Some diseases, such as measles, are most highly communicable before the rash appears and, therefore, before the homemaker may be aware of the disease. The doctor will need to tell the home nurse how the germs of the particular disease are spread and what regulations are required by the health department. To take care of a patient with a communicable disease at home:

1. Assemble all the equipment needed for use every day. This should be at hand so the home nurse will not need to leave the room until she has completed giving care to the patient. Use a washable bedspread. An extra blanket is better than an elaborate quilt since it is more easily washed.

2. Wear a cover-all apron when giving care to the patient. A hook or standard of some sort on which to hang the apron should be provided near the door.

3. Wash the hands before caring for the patient and after giving care before touching anything outside the sickroom.

4. Use clean newspapers or other material in the room for protection of the floor and furniture. A supply of paper towels, paper napkins, and plenty of paper tissues for the patient's use will be convenient and save the home nurse's time and energy.

5. Bring in the bedpan, bedpan cover, and urinal if necessary; keep them out of sight—the closet is a good place.

6. Keep visitors, children, and pets out of the sickroom until the doctor gives his permission for the patient to see them.

When there is a communicable disease, infectious body discharges must be carefully destroyed. Discharges carrying infection will differ depending on the nature of the disease. For example, in tuberculosis of the lungs or in whooping cough, the discharges from the nose and throat must be safely destroyed. In typhoid fever, the discharges from the bowel will carry infection; the safe disposal of these will involve the use of special disinfectants prescribed by the doctor. In addition, all articles soiled with discharges or in contact with the patient must be thoroughly cleansed or destroyed. The home nurse must remember:

1. To burn or otherwise safely dispose of all paper tissues or dressings from the sickroom as soon as possible.

2. To wash thoroughly in hot soapy water, scald, and drain dry all dishes, glasses, or other articles used by the patient.

The home nurse must be particularly careful in taking off and hanging up her apron to fold it so that the outside of the apron, which is contaminated, does not touch her dress, which is *clean,* and to avoid touching with her contaminated hands the inside of the gown, which is considered clean and comes next to her clean dress. Paper gowns can be purchased, but washable cover-all aprons with short sleeves will do just as well. Keep a supply available for frequent changes.

Serving Meals

The home nurse must often cook and care for both the family and the patient. After the patient has eaten, the home nurse should place the soiled paper napkins and leftover solid food in a container, to be burned later, and should pour leftover liquid food into the toilet or waste pail. Food from the sickroom should be disposed of promptly and never shared with others.

When a patient has finished his meal, the home nurse removes the tray with the dishes and utensils to the kitchen; puts them directly into hot, soapy water; and thoroughly washes them, rinsing them in scalding water and letting them drain dry. Dishes and utensils may be left on the tray for the next meal if desired. The doctor will indicate if he feels additional precautions are needed.

Care of Soiled Linen

If soiled linen is sent to a commercial laundry, it should be placed on newspapers on the floor, rolled up, and wrapped in clean wrapping paper or placed in a clean laundry bag marked "Communicable Disease."

If washed at home, soiled linen should be prepared as here suggested, carried to the home laundry tubs, dropped at once into hot soapy water (unless stained), and kept there until washed as usual. This linen should be dried in the sun or ironed. The doctor or the health department regulations may require the use of a special disinfectant.

Linen stained with blood or body discharges should be immersed in cold water before washing with hot soapy water. It is well to become acquainted with methods of removing other stains. For instance, a fruit or vegetable stain is best removed by pouring boiling water over the soiled part, which is held tightly over an open receptacle.

Care of the Bedpan and Urinal

If a bathroom is not available the contents of the bedpan and urinal may be emptied into a covered waste pail. Rinse these articles first in cold water and then wash with hot soapy water; rinse after each using. After emptying waste into the toilet, the waste pail should receive a thorough cleansing with hot, soapy water at least once a day. The doctor will order any special disinfection that may be necessary or will instruct the family if the waste should have special treatment before being put into the toilet.

Cleaning the Sickroom

If possible, a set of cleaning equipment should be kept in the room for use during the illness. An oiled duster, an oiled dust mop, and a small broom and dustpan or a dampened cloth for daily cleaning will be all that are needed if the patient is sick a short time and goes to bed in a clean room. Following illness, the equipment should be cleansed thoroughly and sunned.

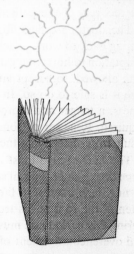

Direct sunlight will help disinfect a book.

Terminal Cleanup

When the period of isolation is over and the patient has recovered, he should have a warm tub bath, a shampoo, and a complete set of clean clothes before being moved to a clean room. The sickroom should be thoroughly cleaned and allowed to air.

1. Hot water and soap should be used whenever possible. The use of a special antiseptic is unnecessary unless especially advised by the doctor.

2. Articles such as the mattress, pillows, cushions, or heavy rugs should be sunned in the open air for about 6 hours.

3. All glass, china, eating utensils, and articles used for treatments should be washed in very hot soapy water, rinsed with scalding water, and allowed to drain dry.

4. Books and toys that cannot be washed should be sunned for several hours. The books should be opened with the pages toward the sun, and they should then be put aside for 2 to 4 weeks. If any of them are library books, the librarian should be notified of the contamination.

THE CONVALESCENT PATIENT

When any sick person begins to get well, he is convalescing. Getting well may be a matter of days or it may take weeks or years, depending upon the nature of the illness and the patient's ability to cope with it. There are some important points for the home nurse and the family to understand about convalescence, for good care during this period speeds the recovery of the patient—mental as well as physical.

The doctor's orders about getting up, eating, sleeping, exercise, and getting back to work or school must be followed. There is always a great temptation to hurry the getting-well process, to stay up just a little longer than allowed, to accept an invitation to a party or go back to work before it is safe to do so. In the case of older persons and after prolonged illness, a longer and more gradual period for increasing activity will be required. Relapses or complications with lasting injury to the body may result from disobeying the doctor's orders during convalescence.

The home nurse must realize that the patient who has been sick for some time is not his usual self. He may be fidgety, irritable, or moody, and he may lack interest in life and refuse food. Weakness and boredom are often at the root of his trouble. The home nurse must be understanding during this period and must try to find a middle course between coddling and overencouragement of the patient.

Home may not always be the best place in which to get well. A fresh scene, freedom from family and business cares, and a change in climate may work wonders for patients who have been sick a long time. The doctor may order such a change in environment. Many hospitals now have their own divisions for convalescent patients, or the public health nurse will be glad to suggest suitable convalescent homes if this seems desirable. Find out whether the convalescent home offers the necessary facilities to continue the treatments ordered by the doctor, for example, a diet for persons with diabetes.

When the patient is convalescing at home, it is especially necessary for the home nurse to recognize the signs of fatigue and to insist on rest before the patient undoes the care of weeks. Signs of fatigue may show during a treatment, when receiving visitors, when sitting up and getting about for the first time, or toward the end of the day. The remedy is to put the patient to bed, give him a warm drink and exclude visitors, thus encouraging him to sleep. After a long or serious illness, much harm can be done by letting a patient get overtired. He will often try not to show fatigue and even deny feeling tired or weak. Children may insist they "feel fine" and may even appear so, though they are really overexcited and still weak.

The usual signs of overfatigue are restlessness, wandering attention, loss of interest in what is going on or being said, pallor, yawning, an increased pulse rate, a slight rise in temperature, a feeling of faintness, or fainting. Later signs are sleeplessness, loss of appetite, and loss of weight.

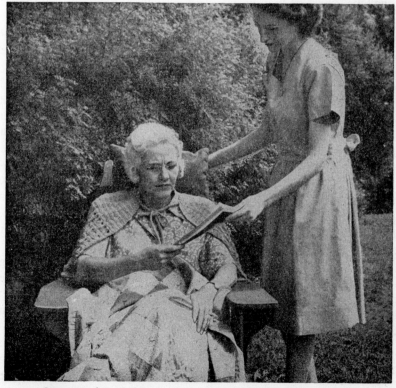

Sitting in the garden sunshine gives variety to patient's day.

Aids to Convalescence

To help the patient recover, the home nurse should:

1. Remove all reminders of illness from the room.

2. Rearrange the furniture or provide different furniture, if advisable and possible; add plants and flowers.

3. Provide fresh clothing, bedclothing, and furnishings.

4. Encourage the patient to resume his usual responsibilities such as dressing, bathing, and eating with the family gradually but steadily.

5. Support the patient's weak muscles by supplying proper chairs and cushions, and shoes in preference to slippers. Exercise should be taken gradually, especially stair climbing. No heavy lifting, stretching, or outdoor sports should be permitted until allowed by the doctor.

6. Get the patient outdoors as soon as possible, weather permitting.

7. Supply appropriate diversions, seeking help from an occupational therapist if the patient is facing a long convalescence. Diversions and occupations should be both purposeful and suited to the individual's interests and abilities.

8. Allow few visitors at first, encouraging more visits as the patient grows stronger.

Return to Work or School

The doctor will usually indicate when the time has come to return to work or school. A patient often wants to return to work before he is really well to avoid losing more time and money. Too early a return to work may mean a serious setback that may cost far more money than another week of absence from work. Half-time work may be feasible as a first step toward regular hours. If children are not completely recovered and able to stay at school full time, it is better to keep them at home unless plans have been agreed upon between the school and parent. Neither employer nor teacher wants a half-sick person on his hands, and it is unfair to the others who may be handicapped by a slow worker or student.

Occasionally after a long illness or injury a patient dreads returning to work or school and keeps putting it off. He may need considerable pushing to get started. If the effort to escape work or study continues too long, consult the doctor. There may be a mental or emotional condition that must be handled with understanding and skill.

What To Report to the Doctor

The home nurse should record the following information about the convalescent patient:

1. The amount of time the patient sat up or walked about.
2. The amount of sleep.
3. The temperature if the doctor has requested it.
4. Food and liquids taken, bowel movements, and general condition.
5. Patient's interests and activities.

THE AGING AND CHRONICALLY ILL

The care of the members of the family who are advanced in age is one of the most common and most demanding duties of the home nurse. Furthermore, there is frequently a close relationship between advanced age and chronic illness. It is, therefore, important for home nurses, particularly those who are young, to understand the special problems outlined in this section.

With advancing years certain changes take place throughout the whole body. There is a general slowing down of all mental and physical powers; the arteries may harden; the bones grow more brittle; and the muscles become less flexible. But so gradually do these changes appear that both the individual and his family may be unaware of them. A person who is unable to meet the physical and mental problems of old age is said to be senile. There is no fixed time when one can be said to have reached the senile state. In general, one whose family history indicates a longer than average life expectancy, whose health has been good, who has been adequately nourished, and who has had regular habits will usually retain his vigor longer than the person who has lived under opposite conditions. Generally, physical vigor and enjoyment of living are the reward for the one who, through the years, has been able to meet successfully the physical and emotional problems of life.

Many people—indeed the vast majority—proceed confidently and cheerily into old age and maintain their alertness and interest in life to its end. Everyone knows crippled, handicapped, even bedridden friends who are the happiest people in the world, who have hobbies of absorbing interest, or who go right on enriching their communities by productive work and volunteer activities after old age is reached. Such people should not be treated as invalids. To be needed and to serve a worthwhile purpose in life is important to the older person. Often limitation of physical activity is compensated for by spiritual growth.

Planning for Old Age

Financial Security. The wise man plans during his earning years for his future and that of his family. Most of the dread of old age stems from fear of poverty, dependency, and physical helplessness or loneliness. While there is no guarantee against the hazards of life, a plan for economic security on retirement is all-important to anyone's peace of mind.

Health Security. Our bodies will wear out. No one has discovered a cure for age, but doctors know many ways of prolonging physical activity, preventing handicapping illnesses, and relieving chronic conditions to the extent that it is entirely possible to live a satisfying life and to escape serious discomfort. A yearly visit to the doctor for a general checkup after the age of 40, additional visits when symptoms of illness appear, and honest observance of the doctor's suggestions will do much to make the advancing years enjoyable. There is almost no excuse these days for suddenly discovering the presence of a chronic illness that has probably been sending out warning signals for the last several years.

Pleasure in Retirement. Retirement, psychologists say, should come whenever decreasing physical or mental power makes it impossible to carry a productive job. They believe retirement should not be an automatic measure imposed on all persons at a specified age, but should be a selective, individual matter. It is natural that those who have led active lives should continue to do some kind of work. It is important also, when retirement is reached, that each of us retire *to* something—some absorb-

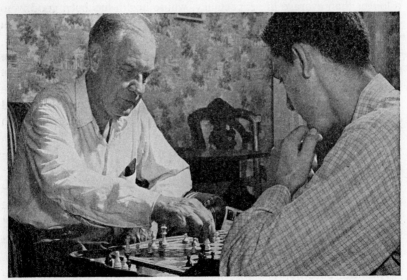

Interest in a hobby and participation in family recreation help prevent loneliness for grandfather.

ing interest, hobby, or suitable activity that will take the place of the daily responsibilities we have left behind. Suggestions for diversions will be found in the reading list on p. 224. An early plan for a retirement activity should be made, as this will usually result in a satisfactory mental adjustment.

Mental Changes

Age and illness may bring decided changes in one's personality and disposition. The man of keen intellect may become childish, absent-minded, and irresponsible; the even-tempered, thoughtful, happy mother may become an irritable, selfish, and moody grandmother. Occasionally these mental changes are so serious that institutional care must be sought for the sake of the safety and happiness of the younger members of the family. In managing these patients at home, it is well to remember that their care resembles that needed by little children, although they must never be treated as children; they need simple food, warmth, regular habits of cleanliness and toilet, freedom from worry and nagging, and easy tasks to occupy their hands. They must be given protection at night and guarded from accidents. They should not be left alone for long.

Elderly people are often as troubled by the evidences of the slowing down of their mental processes as they are by their stiffening bones and muscles. Failure to remember names, dates, and, especially, recent occurrences troubles them. It is not possible to keep as many things in mind as formerly, and occasionally something really important slips by. Much of the slower thinking is to be expected, but psychologists now advise people not to give in to accepting this sort of fumbling but to try to remember, to keep the mind active and busy. Memory failure may be one of the first symptoms of true senility. But if it is not, then it is a bad habit and should be vigorously handled by doing memory exercises, such as reading something and then telling someone what has been read.

The Nature of Chronic Illness

Chronic illness is found in all age groups and is not restricted to people of middle and old age. Studies of illnesses of various types indicate that more than half the chronic illness was among those under 45 years of age. Among the conditions that may afflict young people and lead to prolonged convalescence or a chronic state are heart disease, cerebral palsy (paralysis resulting from a lesion within the skull), rheumatic fever, poliomyelitis (inflammation of the gray substance of the spinal cord), and diabetes; older people may suffer from any one of these as well as kidney disease, arthritis, hardening of the arteries, cancer, and cerebral hemorrhage (bleeding within the skull). Some of the latter diseases also strike the young. Mental illness is often thought of as chronic and usually does require a long period to cure.

The causes of chronic illness are numerous. Physical injury may handicap a person for life, and the infectious diseases sometimes leave conditions that are long in disappearing or may last a lifetime. The infirmities of old age may be sufficiently crippling to be chronic and sometimes incurable.

It is true that many homes throughout our land shelter an aged or chronically ill member of the family—someone not sick enough to need hospital care or feeble enough to require a fulltime hired attendant at home. The care of such persons is frequently a distressing problem to the younger members of the family and can become so serious a burden as to break down the health of the home nurse and disrupt the whole life of the family. At times situations develop in which it is only fair to the rest of the family to seek a place where the chronically ill or incapacitated patient may be properly cared for outside the home. Other means of relieving the home situation are:

1. The various members of the family can help share the burden of caring for the patient and thus give the home nurse opportunity for needed rest and relaxation. If the illness is not communicable, younger members of the family can contribute by helping keep the patient entertained and giving the personal care which does not require the services of the home nurse herself. Joining a home nursing class and learning the easiest and best way to care for an invalid will help avoid uncertainty and worry and save many steps.

2. The employment of a practical nurse or attendant on a full- or part-time basis or as a relief during vacations for the home nurse. (When in need of a registered or practical nurse, consult your family doctor, the official Nurses Registry, the Visiting Nurse Association, or the local health department.)

3. Assistance from the visiting or public health nurse to give the necessary nursing care and treatments as ordered by the doctor once or twice a week and to supervise the home care given. The public health nurse can put you in touch with many types of aids to make home care easier and will plan with you to relieve you of the burden of difficult nursing treatments ordered by the doctor. Charges for visits from these professional nurses are moderate and adjusted to your circumstances. If this community service is available, you should feel free to use it.

Special Needs of the Aging and Chronically Ill

The chronically ill or aged person especially needs the following protections:

1. *Protection from cold:* Feeble and old people feel the cold much more than the strong and active. It may be necessary to supply extra heat in the invalid's room (70° to 78°) and to provide woolen underclothing and wraps when he is in the rest of the house. Drafts from windows must be cut off by screens. Extra blankets, bedsocks, bedjackets, a nightcap, and a hot water bag may be needed on cold nights. Many old people find great comfort in the use of flannel nightgowns and flannel sheets instead of cotton. Old people may develop respiratory diseases such as bronchitis, influenza, and pneumonia, because their resistance is likely to be low. They are usually slow in overcoming even mild infections. Protecting them from exposure and chilling, keeping them well nourished, and getting them out in the sunshine as often as possible will help safeguard them against illness.

2. *Protection from accidents:* Elderly persons do not always see or hear as well as the young, and their muscular reactions are slower. Consequently, extra precautions are necessary to prevent falls, which are a common cause of home accidents. Rugs should be anchored securely (*see* p. 133), and furniture should be sturdy enough to provide safe support when leaned upon or grasped. Stairs should be well lighted and fitted with handrails; the slippery bathtub should be made safe by a rubber suction mat and a handhold; and the use of any new appliance coming into the house should be carefully explained. Icy sidewalks should be avoided in winter. Some of the conveniences the elderly may want for their safety and comfort are a flashlight or a night light in the bathroom, the hall, on the stairs, and in the bedroom; a commode in the bedroom for use at night; rubber-soled shoes; and a stool beside the tub or a bath seat on which to sit in the bathtub if getting in and out of the tub is difficult.

3. *Protection from dependence:* The elderly and chronically ill usually dislike being dependent on others, though occasionally just the reverse is true. The home nurse should encourage the spirit of independence just as far as safety permits. The invalid should have his own room, if possible, simple duties about the house and yard, choice of clothing, care of his person, and freedom to see his friends alone and to make decisions. Within reason the invalid should be granted small favors, such as being allowed to make himself a cup of coffee at dawn if he wishes it, to use a feather bed if that is what he has always been used to, and to smoke if proper precautions are taken and if the doctor permits it. Protection may

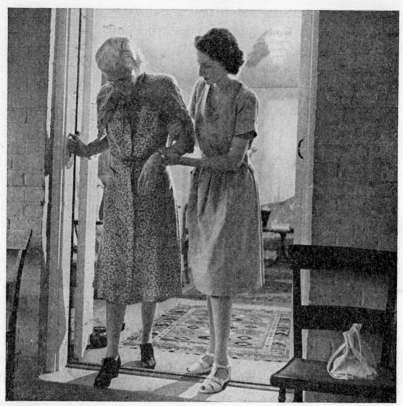

Elderly persons may need special safety devices, such as handholds, built in the home.

have to be offered, but it should be given tactfully. Few persons would wish to prolong their lives if it meant loss of freedom of choice and action. The handicapped person or chronic invalid who faces a succession of monotonous, inactive years needs to develop an interest that will build up his self-confidence and make him feel like a useful person instead of a parasite. Dependent people should be encouraged to learn some occupation that will yield them a little income, if possible. This stimulates self-respect, contributes to a feeling of security, and provides a means of escaping from their troubles.

4. *Protection from loneliness:* Loneliness can be a real and frightening problem affecting the well-being of people at any age, but this is especially true of the elderly person who has retired from active work.

Resources within the individual and his way of life will often influence his ability to entertain himself during later life. Participation in community or family recreational activities, together with making plans to acquire a hobby suited to the physical limitations of the aged, may be a partial answer to the problem.

An enlightened and progressive community will be concerned with providing opportunity for recreational and gainful activities for older persons. The success of such group ventures naturally must depend upon individual participation. The home nurse can encourage such participation when it seems advisable.

When a person has infirmities, such as poor vision or hearing, family members need to be thoughtful about including the aging person in conversation or in interpreting what is being said or done. This may mean that one person at a time should converse with the aged, since the conversation of a group frequently is confusing and tiring.

The home nurse should also keep in mind that one of the best ways of preventing loneliness is to do things for other people. The older person should be given an opportunity to contribute his time and talents to the family group, to friends and neighbors, or to the community whenever conditions make such action possible.

Special Points for the Home Nurse

In caring for the aging and chronically ill, the home nurse should keep in mind the following considerations:

1. *Cleanliness:* Most elderly people dislike and may have less need for frequent baths. This dislike is partly because of the difficulty in using a bathtub and partly because of getting chilled. The home nurse must tactfully suggest partial baths or shower or sponge baths and must offer conveniences for easy bathing—plenty of hot water, a warm room, and safe surroundings. Visits to a beauty parlor or barber shop and to a chiropodist may be welcome.

If the patient is bedridden, a full bed bath twice a week, a partial bath daily, and a daily back rub (*see* The Back Rub, p. 160) are desirable. Special attention must be given to keeping the bed clean, dry, and unwrinkled to prevent bedsores. (*See* Changing the Bed Linen, p. 147.)

Elderly persons frequently suffer from excessive drying of the skin. Sometimes the whole body will need a daily rub with cold cream, cocoa butter, or an oil. If an alcohol rub is given, an oil may be added to it— half rubbing alcohol, half oil (always warmed before use).

It is not easy to keep a bedridden invalid clean and comfortable at all times; yet nothing is so unpleasant to the invalid himself, his family, and his friends as neglect. It is a challenge to the home nurse to make the sickroom a place where people like to come.

2. *Elimination:* Lifetime habits of elimination may change as a person grows older or becomes bedridden. There is often undue concern if the bowels do not move each day, and the patient may be inclined to take cathartics unnecessarily. The doctor will order whatever medicine or diet is suited to the condition. The frequent passing of urine is a very common ailment, and toilet facilities should be available on the same floor as the invalid or at his bedside at night.

If the patient is bedridden, great care must be taken to see that he is cleansed and dried after each use of the bedpan, and if there is no control of the bladder and bowel, the bed will need extra protection, and special efforts must be made to keep the patient clean, dry, and free from bedsores. The use of an air cushion may be essential. Also, the home nurse may pin on the patient a diaper in which a large soft pad of absorbent cotton or cellucotton has been folded. Frequent changes of the diaper are necessary, and attention must be given to the base of the spine and the skin of the buttocks at each change. If he is able to be out of bed, the patient may use a toilet chair during the day—a great help to the home nurse.

3. *Exercise:* The amount of exercise usually will be ordered by the doctor. A certain amount, usually in the form of walking, is beneficial to most elderly persons. A wheelchair will give those unable to walk a change of scene when a car is not available.

Doctors nearly always prefer to have the patient get out of bed and move around as much as possible. Even if this is a painful, slow process and is not desired by the patient, it is often a most beneficial treatment because it keeps the muscles of the legs and back in better condition, relieves pressure on the tissues, and improves the circulation. Also, whether he will admit it or not, it is much better mental hygiene for the invalid to be up and making an effort to act normally. Such exercise usually leads to better sleep. (*See* Helping the Patient from the Bed to a Chair and Back into Bed, p. 154.)

It is often difficult for the home nurse to handle completely or partially paralyzed persons alone. It is often utterly impossible for them to help themselves, to help lift their bodies, or to hold anything. Sometimes even the muscles of swallowing are not under control. The home nurse must have help with patients in this condition unless they are children or adults light enough for the home nurse to handle. If paralyzed from the waist down, the patients can do a good deal to help by using their arms. By providing overhead bars with rope loops to pull on, nearly all these patients can move themselves from side to side as well as up off the bed sufficiently for the home nurse to place the bedpan. The overhead bar must be absolutely secure.

The home nurse must take great care to see that the patient's position in bed is changed frequently. Change of position is important for two reasons: It relieves pressure on the tissues, thus preventing bedsores, and it stimulates the general blood circulation. The home nurse should turn a helpless patient from one side to the other at intervals and should provide adequate support for the body.

4. *Diversions:* Some regular light occupation around the house and garden, a hobby, visitors, and the radio will be found to contribute to the contentment of the elderly and incapacitated. They like recognition and praise for what they accomplish just as others do. Suggestions for diversions that are suitable for them may be found in books at the public library, or advice may be obtained from the occupational therapist (a person who treats diseases by means of prescribed work) at the nearest large hospital or from the public health nurse.

The chronically ill and elderly, especially if they are "roomfast" but not seriously ill, enjoy small parties and surprises. Some of the ways in which the family can provide diversion and untold enjoyment for the invalid are through observance of birthdays and holidays, special meals,

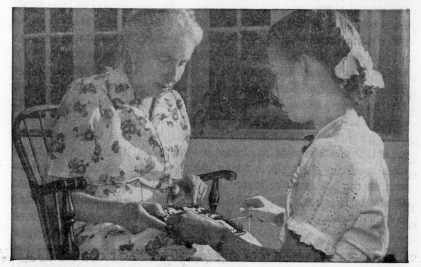

Grandmother feels more a part of the family when her advice is needed.

decorated trays, invitations to two or three friends for a meal, and arranging for the invalid to invite members of the family to dine in his room. Another source of great pleasure to invalids of all ages is a radio within reach at all hours.

Children of school age who are to be in bed several months should be given every opportunity to keep up with their school work. In large cities, the public schools supply visiting teachers, and there are some nursing homes for bedfast children that make it a point to teach the children in classes. Lacking these, it is frequently possible to find someone to come in and teach the lessons supplied by the schools.

Under certain conditions state schools or institutions will be most appropriate places for care. Advice as to their use should be sought from the doctor. Special schools may be advised for the deaf, blind, or spastic child, while special classes in school may take care of the hard-of-hearing, visually handicapped, or crippled child.

Nearly all authorities agree that the feeble-minded child with marked behavior problems should be placed in an institution, especially if there are other children in the family.

Daily Schedule of Care

With a bedridden invalid in the home, it is essential for the peace of the household and the peace of mind of the home nurse to make a plan for smooth accomplishment of all the nursing and housekeeping duties. The invalid whose care is scheduled according to this sort of plan is not likely to have any important part of his care neglected, and the home nurse is less fatigued. She saves herself steps, and by planning ahead is not in a flurry when unexpected duties arise. Try to make a long-range nursing plan as well as a daily plan, which will include the occasional duties along with those to be carried out each day. For example, once a month the home nurse may wish to have the entire sickroom cleaned, aired, and changed about. This may mean moving the patient to another room for a few hours, and for this the help of others will probably be needed. Occasionally she must plan for the patient's shampoo and in the meantime keep the scalp and hair clean by gentle brushing. The mattress on the bed must be turned and the blankets and pillows aired in the sun once a week, if possible. Regular visits from the doctor should be anticipated.

Rehabilitation

The process of restoring as much activity and as many outside interests to the chronically handicapped person as possible has become a real science. The kind and amount of activity and the place where it is carried on all become important both psychologically and physically. An important aim of the home nurse is to prevent needless disability. Thousands of handicapped persons—those crippled by accidents, the mentally ill, the deaf and blind, those born with defects, and, by far the largest group, the chronically ill—must often be cared for at home. This places a responsibility upon the home nurse to help find ways and means of developing self-reliance on the part of the patient in so far as his condition allows. Frequently the home nurse, in caring for members of her own family, is tempted to overprotect or indulge the patient and so delay recovery. It is usually best for the home nurse to seek expert advice about suitable constructive activity for a chronic or handicapped invalid, just as she will want to be sure that all the available known resources for physical rehabilitation are being used, such as body massage, diathermy (treatment to produce heat in the body tissue by means of an electric current), corrective exercises, and light and heat baths. Physical therapy (treatment of diseases by the use of light, heat, water, or air) has been known to work miracles when used under prescribed conditions. Some of these treatments are available in doctors' offices, and most of them in hospital clinics.

Special Appliances. Special appliances such as crutches, braces, belts, trusses, back supports, artificial limbs, or hearing aids may be ordered by the doctor to help the patient lead as normal a life as possible despite his disabilities.

Constant improvements in models and the more common use of such appliances has resulted in a more philosophic acceptance of them by both patients and the public. To achieve the greatest benefit and comfort for the patient, appliances must be selected and adjusted with care. This may, in some instances, require experimentation with different models or readjustment at periodic intervals.

The doctor, nurse, or technician will assist and supervise the patient as he learns to use the devices ordered for him, but the home nurse will need to be alert to see that the patient continues to use them according to instructions. For instance, in the use of crutches she must make sure that the rubber tips are on securely to prevent slipping and that the patient does not place his weight on the underarm rests but supports it through his hands and wrists to prevent injury to the nerves in the arm pit. She will also need to watch for any apparent injury to the patient, such as chafing or swelling, and report this to the doctor.

What To Report to the Doctor

Although visits to and from the doctor may not be frequent for elderly and chronically ill patients, contact with him should be maintained and periodic medical examinations given. The doctor will want the home nurse to report any change in the patient's condition, including loss of appetite or sleep, the presence of a cold or cough (it is especially important to report a persistent or painful cough), sudden loss or gain in weight, bleeding from any part of the body, a lump in any part of the body, inability to pass urine or pain on passing it, spells of dizziness, vision disturbances, or thickness in speech. If the patient is bedridden, notify the doctor at once of any break in the skin, numbness, swelling of the joints, or swelling (puffiness) of the skin at any point.

CARE OF THE DYING

When it is evident to the doctor that the patient is approaching the end of his life, he will usually tell a member of the family. The approach of death and death itself represent a decisive change in family relations. This book does not attempt to give information on means of family adjustment to such a situation. The family as a whole will recognize that spiritual and emotional comfort are particularly needed at this time. The following information is presented to enable the home nurse to give practical aid to the patient and members of the family.

Usually a period of coma or semiconsciousness precedes death, but the family and friends should be reminded that the patient may be able to hear and understand what is going on around him even if he cannot respond to questions. The sense of hearing is often the last sense to be lost, and nothing should be said in the patient's presence to annoy or frighten him. Whispering may be as disturbing as giving way to grief.

A few simple things should be done for the comfort of the patient:

1. There should be quiet and order in the sickroom, and it should be well lighted and aired. Too many visitors may disturb the patient as well as use up the oxygen in the room; however, the patient should not be left alone.

2. The temperature may rise as death approaches, and the patient may feel warm even though his hands and feet are cold. Cover lightly; it is not necessary to use hot water bags.

3. The lips should be kept moist and the mouth and nostrils free from mucus (thick, slippery secretion of the mucous membrane); this can be done by gently wiping out the mouth with cotton swabs dipped in ice water, lubricating the lips with cold cream, and keeping the head raised

on a pillow to ease breathing. The face may be turned to one side and the jaw pushed gently forward to facilitate swallowing the mucus that gathers in the throat. Food or liquids should not be given unless the patient asks for them.

As life ebbs there is less physical care that can be given the patient, and the home nurse should be mindful of the other members of the family who may be too distressed to be aware of their own needs; this is especially true of food and rest. She can reassure them that death is usually kindly, nearly always painless, and often like falling asleep. What may appear distressing for the patient frequently occurs after the patient is no longer conscious. Some patients, however, may be fully aware of the approaching end, are calm and at peace, and wish the loving presence of the family.

After death, the body should be cleansed, the dressings replaced, the hair brushed, a fresh gown (or sheet) put on, dentures, if used, replaced, and a bandage tied under the chin and over the head to keep the jaw from dropping. The eyes may be gently closed. Fresh sheets should be placed under and over the body and a protecting pad placed under the buttocks in case there are discharges from the relaxed bowel and bladder. The undertaker will take care of other procedures.

If the doctor is not present at the time of death, he should be notified at once, as the death certificate must be signed by a physician.

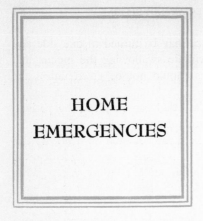

HOME EMERGENCIES

6

DANGER IN SELF-TREATMENT

THERE is a tendency for people to try to treat themselves when sickness occurs. Symptoms may seem slight and too unimportant for medical advice. Sometimes it is inconvenient to see a doctor. It seems much easier to go to the medicine cabinet and select a patent medicine, to stop at the drug store and ask for a remedy, or to take a friend's advice. In accidents also the idea that first aid is sufficient or that someone other than a doctor can tell what is wrong may prove a costly mistake. Obviously, the doctor cannot be summoned for every little ache or pain, but it is important for the homemaker to learn to recognize symptoms, especially those that recur or those that are characteristic of an illness that may be present in epidemic form.

The hazards of self-treatment on the advice of anyone but a doctor may be summarized as:

1. Delay in obtaining the correct treatment.

2. Risk in taking the wrong treatment or medicine, thus making the condition worse or actually producing new and more serious symptoms.

3. Danger of hiding the signs that make it possible for the doctor to diagnose the condition promptly.

4. Waste of money in experimenting with medicines recommended by a well-meaning friend or other person who has not had medical training—money that would bring better returns if used to provide competent medical attention.

DEFINITION AND PURPOSE OF FIRST AID

First aid is the care given a sick or injured person before the services of a doctor can be obtained. One who knows how to give this care properly is able to assist others when they need help most. The purposes of first aid training are to prevent accidents, to train people to do the right thing at the right time, to prevent additional injury, and to provide proper transportation.

The American Red Cross has developed a practical course in first aid that is offered by its chapters throughout the country. The first aid textbook used in this course may be purchased from any Red Cross chapter for a small sum. It covers in detail the treatment of the common emergencies that one is likely to meet. At least one member of every family should complete the Red Cross course in first aid. The *Red Cross First Aid Textbook* should be kept handy for ready reference.

There are a number of emergency situations that occur in every household. The information in this chapter is not intended as a substitute for a first aid course but merely as a review and help to the home nurse in meeting and preventing common home emergencies.

EMERGENCY AND FIRST AID SUPPLIES

It is unnecessary for a family to keep an elaborately stocked medicine cabinet. Many drugs deteriorate with age and are either useless or harmful after they have stood on the shelf for months. Every family should obtain from the doctor a list of the drugs and first aid supplies that he would prefer them to have. Only those drugs or preparations that are to be used for initial emergency treatment need be in the first aid cabinet. The list may include:

A tube of petrolatum (petroleum jelly)
A roll of adhesive tape
A small box of absorbent cotton
A few packages of finger dressings
A few sterile gauze squares
A few gauze bandages of different widths (or clean white cotton cloth torn in strips)
A pair of scissors
A pair of tweezers
A fever thermometer
A medicine glass
A medicine dropper

Perhaps the doctor will suggest adding medications, such as an antiseptic, a laxative for occasional use, a lotion for the treatment of poison ivy and insect bite, or a headache remedy. Whatever he advises can be used with safety.

It is well to have in the house a hot water bag, an ice bag, an enema bag, and a small rubber ear syringe. These are used in many different types of treatment. They should be kept in a drawer or on a special shelf where it is cool and where they can always be located.

No matter what drugs or medicines are kept on hand for emergencies,

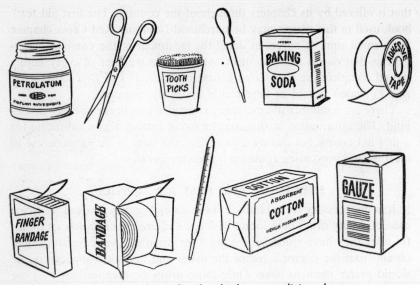

Some essential supplies for the home medicine chest.

they should not be placed in the bathroom cabinet along with toilet articles. Tragic mistakes are frequently made because of confusion regarding bottles. One end of a high shelf in a closet or cupboard (well lighted if possible) should be set aside for medicines and first aid materials.

GENERAL PROCEDURE AT AN ACCIDENT

Here is a simple plan that can usually be followed when accidents occur:

Step 1: Determine whether the victim requires speedy care. Emergency cases are those with severe bleeding, those who have stopped breathing and require artificial respiration, and those in which the victim has received poison by mouth or by injection—for example, the bite of a poisonous snake. In these cases seconds count. A quick glance at the victim and a moment's survey of how the accident happened will usually tell whether one is dealing with an emergency. If so, give immediately the proper first aid as later described. In the great majority of mishaps, however, great speed is not essential; often it is harmful. There is usually time to study the situation, to plan carefully, and to give first aid deliberately.

Step 2: Have the victim lie down; cover him as described under the heading Shock below.

Step 3: Examine the victim carefully.

Step 4: Plan and carry out the necessary procedures.

SHOCK

Shock, a deep disturbance of general body functions, with evidence particularly of disturbed circulation of the blood, may result from any serious injury or deep emotional upset. It may follow immediately or be delayed for some time. Shock opens the way to pneumonia and other serious complications and may lead to death itself. The victim of shock is weak and pale; his skin feels clammy; beads of perspiration may be evident about the upper lip and forehead. Even though these signs may not show up immediately, measures should be taken to combat shock.

The victim should lie flat, preferably in bed. The foot of the bed may be raised from 12 to 18 inches. Provide adequate but not excessive covering, both over and under him, to maintain normal body heat. Avoid overheating or chilling; consider the surrounding temperature. Small amounts of water may be given in most cases. Do not give fluids to an unconscious person or to one who has an abdominal injury, or if it appears that an early operation will be necessary. Handle gently. Pain, bleeding, and rough handling will increase shock.

WOUNDS AND BLEEDING

If the bleeding from a wound is not severe, the first aid worker should apply a dressing to the wound and obtain medical attention. The dressing should be sterile, that is, entirely free from germs. Sterile dressings may be purchased in drugstores and should be at hand in all home or automobile first aid kits. Do not touch the wound, cough over it, or breathe on it. Do not apply ointments, greases, alcoholic liquids, or other so-called home remedies. Never put adhesive or cotton directly on a wound.

Home treatment, even of minor wounds, carries some hazard. The family doctor can advise the method to use. Perhaps he will suggest that the small wound be treated with an antiseptic or carefully washed with clean, preferably boiled, soapy water before a sterile dressing is applied.

In case of a bruise, apply large, cold, wet cloths for a half hour or longer; later apply warm, wet cloths. If several hours have elapsed before any first aid is given, apply the warm, wet cloths at once.

Puncture and Powder Wounds

Allow slight bleeding before applying a sterile dressing. Obtain medical attention at once, because tetanus (lockjaw) may develop in these wounds. Tetanus germs may multiply in almost any wound or burn, but because they grow best in the absence of air, puncture wounds provide good sites for them.

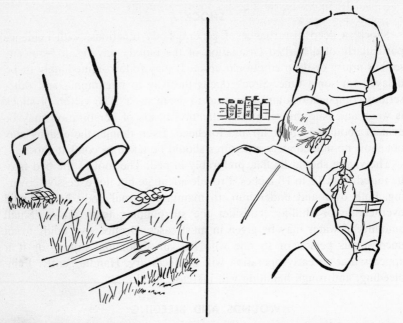

Rusty nails, particularly around barnyards, can cause dangerous wounds. Go to your doctor immediately for protection against infection in case of puncture wounds.

Infected Wounds

Keep the affected part quiet; elevate it slightly on a pillow. Hot, wet packs, using a solution of 3 heaping tablespoonfuls of table salt or 6 tablespoonfuls of Epsom salts to 1 quart of boiled water, are helpful until medical care is available.

Internal Bleeding

Bleeding in quantity from any body cavity requires the immediate services of a doctor. Summon a doctor as soon as possible.

Put the patient to bed, keeping him warm and reassured.

If bleeding seems to be from the lungs or stomach, the patient may have one flat pillow under his head, and the head should be turned to one side; an ice bag may be placed on the chest or stomach. Blood from the lungs is usually frothy and bright red, while blood from the stomach is usually dark red. Crushed ice may be given for thirst.

If the bleeding is from the rectum, vagina, or bladder, keep the patient lying flat, with the foot of the bed elevated from 12 to 18 inches. It is especially important to call the doctor promptly if there is vaginal bleeding during pregnancy.

Avoid moving a patient who is bleeding. Keep him quiet and warm and if possible do not let him see the blood.

Nosebleed

A nosebleed victim should remain sitting, with the head held back. Apply large, cold, wet towels to his face; pinch the nostrils together for a time. Advise him not to cough, walk about, or blow his nose. If bleeding does not stop within 10 or 15 minutes, send for the doctor.

BURNS AND SCALDS

If a burn or scald has merely reddened the skin, sterile petrolatum or any good burn ointment will give relief. If the skin is blistered or more severely burned, apply a sterile dressing, moistened in a baking soda or salt solution (3 tablespoonfuls to 1 quart of warm water), bandage snugly, and obtain medical care. Burns caused by hot liquids are common in the home. Do not attempt to remove the clothing but cut the fabric away from the burn and cover with a moist dressing. Treat severe burn cases for shock, because it is likely to develop.

In case of a chemical burn, wash off the chemical quickly with large amounts of cool water. Then give the same first aid as for other burns. In case the eyes are affected, put a drop or two of castor oil or mineral oil into the eye after washing thoroughly with water. Send for the doctor.

Sunburn

Severe sunburn is dangerous. If it is extensive the person may develop a fever and become quite ill. A severe sunburn may be acquired on a cloudy day, especially at the seashore or on the water.

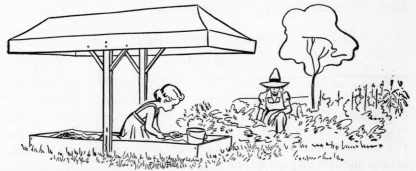

Provide protection from sun's rays. Sunburn can be painful and dangerous.

Snow burn, a deep burn from the reflection of the sun on snow, can be painful, especially to the eyes, and sometimes results in temporary snow blindness. Protect the skin, wear dark glasses, and avoid long exposure. Application of a burn ointment, sweet oil, or cocoa butter before exposure to the sun helps protect the skin and keeps it soft.

First aid care for sunburn and snow burn is the same as for any other burn. For the treatment of eyes affected by the sun, apply cold compresses and consult an oculist (eye doctor).

POISONING

Among children under 14 years of age, poisoning ranks third as a cause of accidental death in the home. Such accidents are usually the result of carelessness on the part of older members of the family in leaving poisonous drugs or chemicals where children can get them. Any drug may be poisonous if taken in large amounts. Children especially are victims of this kind of poisoning.

Persons who swallow poison must be given immediate care. Make the victim drink five or six glasses of fluid to dilute the poison. Baking soda in water, soapy water, salt water, or tap water may be used. Except in the cases listed below, induce vomiting. This may be done by tickling the back of the throat with a finger. Repeat several times, and after the stomach contents have been vomited, give the victim a soothing drink, such as milk, and keep him quiet. Call a doctor.

Exceptions to the treatment described are poisoning by a strong acid, such as arsenic, or a strong alkali, such as lye. *Do not induce vomiting,* because of the danger of perforating the stomach. In case of acid poisoning, give baking soda in water, then milk or egg white. For alkali poisoning, give lemon juice or vinegar, then milk. For strychnine poisoning, dilute with liquids but do not induce vomiting.

LOSS OF CONSCIOUSNESS
Simple Fainting

If a person feels faint, he should lie down or put his head down between his knees. He may be extremely pale and may or may not lose consciousness. Victims of simple fainting revive quickly if they lie flat. When consciousness returns, give hot coffee or tea but do not permit the victim to arise at once. If the victim does not quickly revive, call a doctor, because the case may not be one of simple fainting.

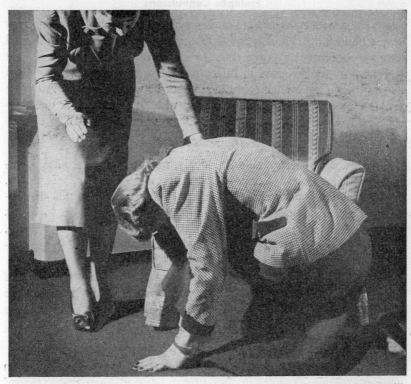

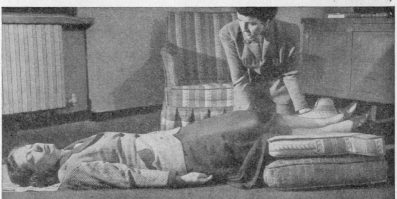

First aid for fainting. *(Top)* Have patient kneel with head down.
(Bottom) Have patient lie down with head lowered.

Epileptic Convulsions

A person with epileptic convulsions may become pale or the skin may have a bluish tinge. He may fall to the ground, become unconscious, and have violent muscular movements. Do not restrain him but try to prevent him from injuring himself in falling against nearby objects. Protect his tongue by placing a stick or wadded paper between his teeth. After the attack is over, allow the person to sleep without disturbing or questioning him.

Convulsions

Convulsions, which come on suddenly, require prompt medical treatment (except epileptic seizures—see the previous description). In adults, convulsions are usually caused by a head injury, some internal disturbance, or an infection such as tetanus (lockjaw) or meningitis. In babies or children, convulsions may be caused by a digestive disturbance, fever, nutritional deficiencies, injury, or infection. Convulsions during pregnancy or delivery are especially serious.

Symptoms of convulsions are muscular twitchings, first of the face and later of the arms and legs or the entire body. The body may become stiff, with the head drawn back; the weight of the body often rests on the head and heels. The face is pale at first and then becomes bluish, particularly about the mouth.

Relief Measures for Adults. Place the patient in a relaxed position wherever he happens to be and send for the doctor. Keep him warm and as quiet as possible. When the convulsion is over, he may be put to bed and kept quiet until the doctor arrives.

Relief Measures for Babies and Children. Place the child in a warm bath. The water should be comfortably warm, tested by the home nurse's elbow. (There is danger of burning the child in the excitement of the moment if the water is not tested.) If preferred, the child may be wrapped naked in a blanket wrung out of warm water, then in a dry blanket to keep the warmth in. (*See* Hot Applications, p. 181.) Both treatments should continue for about 30 minutes. After the bath or pack, give an enema of clear water, or salt and water (1 teaspoonful to 1 pint). When the enema is finished, keep the child quiet in bed until the doctor sees him.

Sunstroke and Heatstroke

The victim of sunstroke or heatstroke has a rapid, full pulse and dry skin. In many instances he becomes unconscious. The face is usually flushed. Remove him to a cool, shady place; take off his clothing, and sponge the entire body with cool water. Do not give stimulants.

Heat Exhaustion

Heat exhaustion results from depletion of salt in the body. Unlike sunstroke, the skin is pale and clammy, instead of flushed and dry. Beads of perspiration appear on the upper lip and forehead, and the eyes are vacant and lack luster. The victim should lie down in a place where air circulation is good and if conscious should be given salt water (1 teaspoon to 1 glass of water) at intervals of 5 to 10 minutes. He should be covered lightly and the doctor called. Loss of consciousness sometimes occurs.

Heart Attack

If the victim's breathing is difficult, elevate his head and shoulders. See that there is no noise, conversation, or unnecessary visiting to disturb him. If he can swallow, give him warm coffee or tea. In certain cases the pain is so great that the patient insists upon walking about. Advise him to be quiet, but do not urge him too strongly. Reassure him tactfully, because fear may be great. The victim of a heart attack may or may not lose consciousness. Call the doctor.

ACUTE ABDOMINAL PAIN

Send for the doctor at once. Do not give medicine, treatment, or food. Put the patient to bed. Small amounts of cracked ice or water may be given for thirst. Never apply heat to the abdominal area except on the orders of a physician.

LEG CRAMPS

In case of cramps in the leg muscles, apply hot, wet towels to the leg and massage the affected part with a liniment or rubbing alcohol. Elevate the leg slightly, bending the knee. If the victim is allowed up, stepping flat on the foot of the affected leg will usually relieve cramps in the calf of the leg and in the foot.

CROUP

Croup usually begins suddenly at night when the child wakens with a hoarse, deep cough, and has difficulty breathing. It may be caused by a cold, but it sometimes develops when there is no evidence of a cold. Since a hoarse, croupy cough is one of the early symptoms of one type of diphtheria, the throat should always be examined carefully when such a cough develops. If the throat is red and has grayish white spots anywhere on it, a doctor should be called at once.

A child who has repeated attacks of croup should be under the doctor's care, so that the condition causing the attacks may be corrected. Building up the child's general health and protecting him from extremes of weather will sometimes help him to overcome the condition.

Relief Measures. The child should be made to vomit so that any mucous plug in the throat may be dislodged. (Ask the doctor what he wants used for this purpose.) Apply either hot or cold compresses to the throat and chest. An ice bag on the throat often brings immediate relief. If a child has a tendency to croup, an ice collar is a wise investment because of its convenience. Inhalations of steam usually give relief. (*See* Inhalations and Throat Irrigations, p. 188.)

BITES

Dog and Cat Bites

In all cases of dog and cat bites or the bites of other animals, such as squirrels, wash the wound freely and gently, using soap and water. Apply a mild tincture of iodine and a dressing. Consult a physician at once, even though the wound seems minor, because of the possible danger of rabies (hydrophobia), a disease that is always fatal. The doctor can give injections that, if started soon enough, will prevent rabies. In the case of a dog bite, tie up the dog and place it under the observation of the local health department. Dogs that have been infected with rabies may seem to be perfectly well at first, but always die within 2 weeks.

Poisonous Snake Bites

The victim of a bite by a poisonous snake should be kept absolutely quiet. Immediately fasten a tight band around the affected arm or leg just above the bite. Make several cuts at least ¼ inch deep around the wound and apply suction to draw out the venom, using a suction cup or the mouth. The poison, if swallowed, is not harmful. Treat for shock and transport the victim with care to a hospital or doctor.

Tick Bites

Ticks should be removed carefully to get the entire tick. Heat applied near the tick will often cause it to release its hold. If the head is accidentally left in the skin, try to remove it without crushing it by pressing the fingers against the skin below the area of the bite. Apply a compress moistened with ammonia in water or a paste made of baking soda and cold cream. (A lotion such as calamine may also be used to relieve itching

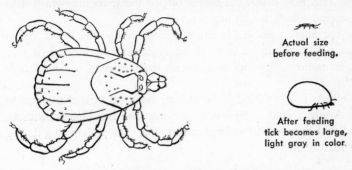

Actual size before feeding.

After feeding tick becomes large, light gray in color.

Learn to recognize ticks. They may transmit disease.

and pain.) Ticks may spread such dangerous diseases as Rocky Mountain spotted fever. If you live, work, or play in regions where ticks are common, consult your doctor concerning vaccination against spotted fever.

FOREIGN BODIES

In the Ear

Foreign bodies in the ear, such as grain, beads, shot, or insects, require the attention of a doctor. Unskilled efforts to remove foreign bodies may only push them farther in and possibly injure the eardrum. Never use hairpins, crochet hooks, or similar instruments to remove foreign bodies from the ear.

If the foreign body is an insect, the following measures may be taken:

1. Have the victim lie on the unaffected side.

2. Drop warm, sweet oil or mineral oil into the affected ear. The insect usually suffocates in the oil and floats to the surface where it can be removed.

3. Have the victim turn over on the affected side so that the oil can drain out. If this treatment does not remove the insect, a doctor should be consulted.

In the Eye

Never rub the eye that has a foreign body (sand, cinder, insect) in it, since this may injure the delicate covering of the eyeball or imbed the object so that it will be difficult to remove. Take these first aid measures:

1. Have the person hold the eyelid closed—lightly—without touching it, so that the tears will accumulate and perhaps wash out the object.

2. Wash the hands and pull the upper lid over the lower one two or three times. This may brush the object off, or the tears may wash it to the inside corner where it can be removed.

3. Press the finger against the cheek directly below the lower lid, so that the inner surface can be seen. If the object can be located, it may sometimes be removed by touching it with the corner of a clean hand-kerchief

If these efforts fail to dislodge the object, make no further attempt to remove it. Apply a cold compress to the eye and bandage it, without pressure, so that the eye will be kept at rest. Take the patient to a doctor for further treatment.

In the Nose

When an insect, grain of corn, or something similar becomes lodged in the nose, a few drops of sweet oil may be dropped in to relieve irritation and help prevent swelling. There is usually no immediate danger from such an accident, but to relieve his discomfort the person should be taken to a doctor to have the object removed as soon as possible. Pending removal, he should refrain from blowing the nose violently or with one nostril held shut.

In the Stomach

Children frequently swallow such objects as coins, pins, tacks, buttons, and safety pins. These may or may not do harm, depending upon the nature of the object. Do nothing in the way of treatment, but call the doctor or take the child to him at once for advice.

In the Throat

Pieces of food, fishbones, nutshells, coins, false teeth, and other similar objects sometimes become lodged in the throat or upper wind-pipe. Although the air passage is not completely closed, the throat may be thrown into a spasm and the patient will be in great distress. His face becomes red or bluish; he gasps for breath and has violent fits of coughing. It is possible for him to collapse from lack of air.

If the object is not too far down in the throat, a quick slap between the shoulders with the head held down will sometimes dislodge it. A child may be lifted up by his feet or placed across a table so that he hangs head down. If this does not dislodge the object, call the doctor without further delay or take the victim to a hospital. If necessary, give artificial respiration *(see* the *Red Cross First Aid Textbook* for information about suffocation and artificial respiration).

EMERGENCY CARE FOR THE BIRTH OF A BABY

Occasionally a baby is born before a doctor or nurse can arrive, or there may be an unavoidable delay in getting to the hospital. Since the birth of a baby is nearly always normal when there is a short period of labor, the home nurse should remain calm. A few things must be done to help safeguard the mother and baby. It will usually be a great help if someone with experience in attending births or even a woman neighbor who has had a baby can be present to assist.

If labor starts and the doctor has been notified, the home nurse should go ahead with the following preparations:

1. Arrange the mother's bed so that the mattress will be well protected by waterproof material or pads made from several thicknesses of paper covered with cloth.

2. Make a warm bed for the baby. A clothes basket, a box lined with a blanket, or a bureau drawer placed on firm chairs or on a table will do. Keep the baby's blankets warm; get out his shirt and diapers and have them warming.

3. Have the mother put on a clean nightgown and, if up and about, a dressing gown, stockings, and slippers.

4. If there is no prospect of having a doctor or nurse present, get ready a pair of sharp scissors for cutting the baby's umbilical cord (cord that connects the placenta with the navel of the baby in the womb). The scissors must be boiled for 10 minutes. At the same time, boil either three lengths of white cotton tape or stout, soft string or three strips of strong muslin cloth ¾ inch wide. At least 14 inches for each length will be needed. (Avoid using hard, thin string as it may cut into the umbilical cord.) Leave the scissors and tape in the basin of boiled water, covered, to cool. Get out a package of sterile gauze dressing, but do not open it. The dressing is used to cover the stump end of the cord after it has been cut.

5. Place close at hand the basin containing the boiled tape and scissors and a basin for washing the home nurse's hands. Have the other things ready for use.

After the baby is born, there are four things that have to be done, and anyone with clean hands and common sense can do them:

1. Pick up the baby carefully, leaving the cord slack and holding him head down. Bend his head back a little so that any mucus or fluid can

run out of his mouth. After the baby is breathing well, to help his heart action, place him on his right side on his own clean blanket which has been placed on top of the blanket that covers the mother. Keep his head lowered to allow the remaining mucus to drain out of his mouth. If the room is cool, cover his body with his own blanket while preparing to take care of the cord.

2. If the doctor has not arrived by this time, get ready to cut the baby's umbilical cord. Remember, this does not have to be done immediately. Take all the time necessary. Bring the gauze dressing and the pan containing the scissors and tape to the bed. Open the dressing without touching the inside. Wash the hands well with soap and water; then take one piece of the tape and tie it tightly around the cord about 6 inches from the baby's body. Tie the other piece of tape tightly 2 inches farther out. With the sterile scissors cut the cord between the tapes. If there is any bleeding from either end, fold back that end of the cord and tie another piece of sterile tape around it. Cover the cut end of the cord with sterile gauze and pin a band around the baby's body just firmly enough to hold the gauze in place.

3. Keep the baby warm and protected at all times. Wrap him in the blanket square and lay him on his right side, head slightly lowered, in his bed. Well-protected hot water bags may be placed at the feet and sides. If there are no hot water bags or other means of keeping him warm, tuck him under the blanket, face uncovered, beside his mother. Be sure to see that he is breathing easily and that there is no bleeding from the umbilical cord.

4. The afterbirth or placenta will be expelled a little later without assistance from the home nurse. Do not pull on the cord. As soon as the afterbirth comes, slide it out on the pad previously placed under the mother's hips or into a basin and wrap it up for the doctor to examine later. The contracted uterus (womb), a hard mass about as big as a large pear, can be located in the mother's abdomen just under the navel. The abdomen must be rubbed or massaged until this firm mass is felt. To prevent hemorrhage, it is important that the uterus remain contracted for the first hour after delivery of the placenta. Repeated massage may be needed to keep it firm. If the mother has lost a great deal of blood, elevate the foot of the bed. The mother should be kept warm and should lie on her back with her legs together. If she seems to have a slight chill, give her a warm drink such as tea, coffee, milk, or bouillon. Wipe her face and hands with a damp towel.

Keep on trying to get the doctor. It is important that he come as soon as possible to treat the baby's eyes, since certain infections may be prevented by prompt treatment. The doctor will also need to examine the mother and baby to be sure everything is all right.

CARE OF THE PREMATURE BABY AT HOME

If the baby is born prematurely at home, the most important thing is to keep him warm and to avoid unnecessary handling. The doctor should be called at once. The less the baby is handled, the better. He should not be dressed—not even diapered—but wrapped loosely in a soft flannel or wool receiving blanket or square, with his face exposed. A soft pad or folded diaper may be placed under the buttocks. He should then be placed in a box, basket, or carton, *well-wrapped* hot water bags or jars of hot water at his sides and feet. If possible, the air surrounding the baby should be as warm as 86 or 88 degrees, but not warmer. Be sure the air is reaching his face. It will not be necessary to feed him until the doctor arrives, unless he cannot get there for 6 to 8 hours. In that case the baby may be fed a small amount of warm (not hot) boiled water, to which a pinch of sugar has been added. Use a medicine dropper for this purpose.

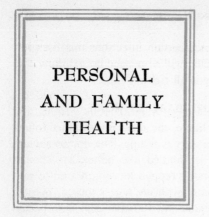

PERSONAL AND FAMILY HEALTH

7

NOT many years ago the word "health" had a much narrower meaning than it now has. We used to think of it as implying physical health only, and we were mainly interested in preventing illness or curing it.

But of late we have been looking at a broader stretch of the world than before, and we have had to broaden our ideas to match this wider horizon. Almost 60 nations have decided, through the World Health Organization, that health is one of the things that is the world's business, and they have set up a new definition of it. From now on it will mean to us not just freedom from disease but a state of mental, social, and emotional health, as well as bodily vigor.

In the home, where personal and family health begins, the home nurse can make a direct contribution to the prevention of illness if she recognizes the need for proper care of every family member. By knowing procedures for care of the baby from the time he gets his start, she can contribute to his becoming a healthier adult.

Throughout this chapter reference is made to various publications prepared by the Children's Bureau, Federal Security Agency, Washington 25, D. C. These include *Prenatal Care,* Publication No. 4 (15 cents); *Infant Care,* Publication No. 8 (15 cents); *Your Child From One to Six,* Publication No. 30 (15 cents); *Your Child From Six to Twelve,* Publication No. 324 (20 cents); and *Guiding the Adolescent,* Publication No. 225 (15 cents). For additional information on mother and child care, consult these publications, which may be available free from your state or local health department or may be purchased from the Superintendent of Documents, Government Printing Office, Washington 25, D. C.

PRENATAL AND MATERNITY CARE

In recent years the number of women who die as a result of giving birth to a child has dropped sharply. This decrease has been largely the result of technical and medical advancements and of the success of efforts to get women to go to a doctor early in their pregnancy. Every woman who not only heeds this advice herself but who also uses her influence among her friends and neighbors to get them to follow this practice is helping to cut down the maternity death rate.

Not only are deaths among mothers fewer when women are under a doctor's care from the start, but many miscarriages, infant deaths, and deaths due to premature birth are also prevented when mothers follow the rules of good hygiene throughout pregnancy and their doctors are able to forestall trouble.

Hesitation about going to a doctor may be caused by any one of several things. The expense looms large in many women's minds, but the practice of many physicians of charging a lump sum for the entire period of prenatal and maternity care should encourage women not to put off getting in touch with their doctor as soon as they suspect they are pregnant.

Hesitation because of fear of the physical examination that will be made is less frequent than it used to be, when false modesty was more common. Acting sensibly now may actually prevent nervous fears later on, for a doctor's measurements and observations help him to know what to anticipate.

Then there are women who just "put off" for no good reason. They forget that the doctor's advice about diet and daily routine, his examinations of urine, and his taking of blood pressure may save them from real trouble, not to mention worry or expense.

It is a great comfort to have a reliable doctor and to feel free to ask any of the little—or big—questions that are bound to arise. No written word can possibly cover all the individual questions, whether before the coming of a first baby or a later one. So much is constantly being added to medical knowledge that even a woman who has borne a child quite recently may find that there are new ways of increasing her comfort and the prospective baby's well-being.

The physician and nurse, either in a private office or in a clinic, are ready to give any kind of help they can. Whether the question is one of finances, caring for other children when the baby is born, or helping to decide whether the birth will take place at home or in the hospital, no question is too unimportant, or too big, to discuss with them.

Having a baby is a whole-family affair. It concerns the father equally with the mother. Particularly at the coming of the first baby, a man and his wife will need to begin to think about and plan for the changes and adjustments in their lives that they can hardly be fully aware of until the baby is actually a living, breathing presence. Thinking ahead of time

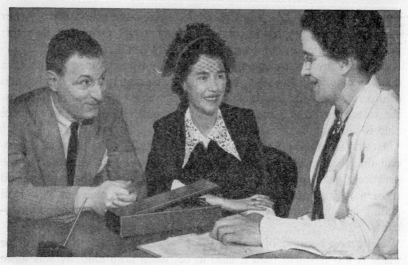

An early visit to the doctor is essential in prenatal care.

about some of the ways in which life is going to be different will make the adjustments easier. Recognizing, for example, that one of them is possibly going to be more "nervous" about the baby, more inclined to be concerned over the slightest cough, or more careful about cleanliness may help parents to realize that they now have a new reason for being generous and understanding of each other's attitudes. The baby will be "their" baby, and yet he is not going to be a possession they can treat as they like. He is "theirs" only in so far as they are mature and sensible enough to see his needs as an individual.

Some of these are among the reasons why it is good to have both prospective parents go when the first visit to the doctor is made, and to attend prenatal discussion groups when they are available.

The parents will want to talk over the problem of where the baby is to be born; if it is to be in a hospital, they may want to inquire about the hospital's policy as to the "rooming-in" plan. In some hospitals the mother will be able to decide whether she prefers to have the baby at her bedside all the time, for part of the time each day, or to see him only at feeding time. Hospitals usually refer to this as "rooming-in." If she has him in the room with her, she can watch how the nurse cares for him and learn a great deal even before she feels strong enough to do much herself.

Fortunately, most mothers are able to breast-feed their babies and thus carry out nature's plan for nourishment for the young infant. However, while a decision to breast-feed may be made before birth, it is not always possible to carry it out. Even the mother who really wants to nurse her baby and who follows her doctor's suggestions as to ways in which she can prepare herself for it may be disappointed. But this should be talked over with the doctor beforehand. He can reassure the parents about ways of making bottle feeding successful.

Parents having their first baby will also want to select at this time the doctor or baby specialist who will care for their baby (if they can afford private care) so that he can become acquainted with the baby from the start.

There will be the question of supplies to think of—those needed for home delivery (if the baby is to be born at home), for the baby himself, and for the mother's use at the hospital. (All are listed in *Prenatal Care,* Publication No. 4, Children's Bureau.) The layette for a baby should be simple. A baby does not enjoy fancy clothes, and he will soon outgrow his first ones. It is well to have the layette on hand by the sixth or seventh month of pregnancy.

The baby's basket or crib may be placed in the parents' room, but after the first few days a baby does not need close watching. His parents may get more rest if he is not in the same room with them, where they listen for every sound. After the first few months he too will sleep better in a room alone.

Along with other preparations for a baby's coming is the need of preparing other children in the family. To tell children about the expected birth too far ahead of time makes the waiting period long. A month or two seems a long time to little children. Even with the most thoughtful preparation there is likely to be some jealousy, though it may not show up in ways that can be thus labeled. Some young children betray their insecure feelings by going back to more babyish ways of acting. Any oddities of behavior in a new baby's brothers and sisters should be considered as possibly the result of their getting less attention than before, and should be treated with patience. It is usually the parents' thoughtlessness or extra busyness that brings about such behavior. It pays to take special pains to give more, rather than less, loving care to other children on the arrival of a new family member. Even though there may be less *time* to give them, the *quality* of the attention may be made to count. A mother can read to an older child while she nurses the baby.

By following her doctor's orders, a woman can usually free herself from fear or worry about complications or about childbirth itself. The less fear a person has, the less difficult the birth is likely to be. Knowing about how the baby is growing, what takes place when he is ready to be born, and how the uterus contracts and relaxes to assist in his birth helps the mother to approach labor calmly and confidently. Her husband can be of great help to her during this period. If he knows what is going on, he will be less apprehensive.

It will be part of the husband's responsibility to make things easy for the new mother when she is up and around again. If help can possibly be afforded, now is the time it is essential. The father himself can be especially helpful—though it is hard—by taking over responsibility during the night. If the mother takes things as easily as she can and refuses to worry over what she can't do, she will be more likely to find that her body is in good condition when she has her final checkup by the doctor 6 weeks after the baby's birth. Unless she has good care after a baby's birth and a leisurely return to her full routine, a mother can hardly be in a state of health that encourages enjoyment of her baby. And a baby whose parents enjoy him will more likely be a happy, contented baby.

THE BABY'S FIRST YEAR

The physical needs of a young baby are few and simple. Food, sleep, warmth, and cleanliness are the first essentials, and help in supplying these will come from your physician or the well-baby clinic doctor. The baby's emotional needs are fully as important. First social responses to loving care come early when he smiles or stops crying when talked to or held. Close personal contact is one of the first ways of contributing to security and happy progress. This has been demonstrated by the poor development of babies in institutions, where little individual care can be given.

The coming of the baby involves many changes in his parents' habits. No longer are they "free agents" with only themselves to think about. But along with the loss of personal freedom there is a gain as the parents take a step toward more mature and responsible adulthood. The coming of the baby gives his parents opportunity for expanding affection through sharing in his care. They develop just as their baby does. A new sense of community responsibility arises as the family is established and begins to be aware of the interplay among home, neighborhood, and larger community group. The parents begin to recognize their need for information about child development in order to meet the changing needs that come with growth.

Fitting the baby into the family involves an easy acceptance of the trial and error period when he is little by little falling into a fairly orderly schedule of eating and sleeping. The mother who fully expects to nurse her baby may by her attitude influence her ability to do so. Even though she may not have quite enough milk for the baby at first, she should not give up. The act of nursing promotes the secretion of milk, and as the baby gets practice in sucking he will help to stimulate a greater flow of milk.

During the first few weeks, when the baby may not stay awake to nurse long at a time, the advantages of having his food "ready," so to speak, at all times, is a particular help to the mother. Before she gets her strength back, and while the care of the baby is new to her, the preparation of a formula and warming bottles whenever the baby is hungry is a good deal of a burden. The problem of having enough bottles prepared to take care of a baby's demands is a considerable one. A baby cannot, of course, be allowed later to finish a bottle that he half-emptied at an earlier feeding. This is because of bacterial growth that is liable to occur in rewarmed milk.

Not only is it simpler and easier to breast-feed a baby, but also a great satisfaction to his mother to feel that she can contribute to her child's well-being in this way. However, if there is some reason why bottle feeding must be substituted, a mother should not feel guilty or worried for formulas can be found that take good care of a baby's needs.

Three- or four-hour schedules were originally advised because experience had proved that regularity in feeding results in healthier babies. But regularity and rigidity are two different things. In their efforts to follow a regular schedule, many mothers watch the clock too carefully, forgetting that the "clock" of the baby's hunger is better to go by. Until he is several weeks old, a baby cannot take into his small stomach enough food to last long, and for the early period of infancy frequent feeding may be necessary. The mother may make mistakes at first and perhaps nurse him or give him his bottle when, if she had waited a few minutes, he would have stopped crying and gone back to sleep. Maybe all he needed was to have his diaper changed or to be turned over in his crib.

Some babies have a way of turning night into day at first, or of making the evening hours their most wakeful ones. Parents who expect irregularity during the first month or two and are not disturbed by it will find that they are gradually managing to fit the baby's needs to their own requirements and habits. To parents with their first baby, everything is so new that they feel a good deal of uncertainty. They need the comfort of knowing that everyone goes through this and that their own good sense will often be a sound guide. Each baby is an individual, so bringing up the baby by "the book" is an impossibility.

Having a competent physician will contribute not only to the baby's well-being but also to his mother's peace of mind, and therefore will promote more relaxed feelings about his care. Immunization and advice about disease prevention may be obtained through regular visits to the doctor's office or to the well-baby clinic. By following the suggestions on infant care, the mother can judge when it is necessary to call the doctor and what to do until he comes. Learning the symptoms that make isolation desirable will help to keep the other children's colds or other infections from endangering the baby.

The baby's physical growth will be greatest in the first year. He will probably double his weight in 6 months and triple it by the end of the first year. Along with growth in size comes development of mind and muscles. The time of reaching each stage of achievement will be different for each baby, but the development follows a regular order: first the smile; then the uttering of sounds and holding up his head. Next comes the ability to grasp something with his hands and, shortly, the power to roll completely over from back to stomach. Sitting up alone comes next; then creeping or crawling. The stages that go before walking are also orderly: first, pulling himself to a standing position; then walking by holding on to something; then standing alone; and, finally, taking several steps alone.

In order for the baby to have the best opportunity for developing his capacities, his surroundings and schedule must be planned for maximum freedom. In early infancy he needs plenty of chances to kick and stretch unclothed, to be frolicked with, to be sung to. As he grows, his physical surroundings must be kept free from danger. His bed and play pen, for example, should be painted with nonpoisonous paint. A safe place should be provided where the baby may crawl and climb, where there are no small objects to be swallowed, no sharp edges to cause bruises. When he stands or walks alone, loose objects will need to be put out of reach so that he can explore and experiment safely.

The baby's emotional life unfolds steadily. A baby has no inborn fears, and if his parents are careful they can prevent many from arising. Using care when the baby is bathed so that he does not slip or get water splashed in his face will help keep bath time happy. Anger will appear when a baby is frustrated, so the fewer and milder the frustrations, the fewer the outbursts of temper. A baby whose hunger and other needs are satisfied with reasonable speed will have few occasions for anger. Dressing and undressing are frustrating—any constraint is—so they should be done quickly. The need for simple clothing is obvious.

The baby whose needs are understood and attended to promptly is being given the foundation for a happy, relaxed personality and an orderly emotional development. His parents' expressions of affection, their enjoyment of him, will be reflected in his responses and behavior.

What the baby learns is dependent on his parents' manner and attitudes; if they are too eager to see him develop, he will feel the pressure and put up resistance. "Wait for nature" might be a watchword for parents. Why begin trying to train a child to keep dry until his nervous system has developed enough to make possible some control on his part? Why, on the other hand, keep him from learning to feed himself just because it is a messy business at first?

Patience, more patience, and humor will help when any learning is taking place. When a child is ready he will learn; before that, no amount of urging or prodding will do any good. During eating, the mother who is relaxed, confident, and unhurried will have a coöperative child. When food refusals occur, she will pass over them lightly, trying again later on. She will encourage her baby to use a spoon by giving him semi-solids, like mashed potatoes, to begin on. She will let him have his bottle as long as he wants it, but will offer him fruit juices and milk from a cup early, so that he may have a chance to get used to it. She won't insist on his finishing a meal when he is too tired.

Learning to sleep at suitable times and places should be a natural procedure, but the mother can help by making the conditions right. Often arrangements for the baby to be in a room alone are difficult but rearrangements that make it possible will pay off in a baby free from tenseness.

Learning to control bowel movements and to keep dry will have only a slight place late in the first year's routine. If the mother begins to notice some degree of regularity in the times of movements or wetting, she may take advantage of them. But to expect any real toilet training so early is to be disappointed. Coöperation on the child's part will be endangered by anything approaching a determined effort. When the child is ready, he will learn speedily, but he may not be ready for many months.

The parents of a baby have two goals in mind: first, a healthy, happy baby who enjoys and is enjoyed by his family; and second, a baby who is progressing from complete helplessness to some degree of self-reliance and ability to adjust to others. He must face some restrictions, like not being allowed to play with grandfather's glasses. But the restrictions must be fitted to his abilities; for example, he should not be expected to sit quietly on the toilet for a long time.

Warm, responsive, understanding parents will be looking for and expecting changes, and by so doing will not fall into a cut-and-dried pattern that does not allow for growth.

THE PRESCHOOL YEARS

A noticeable slowing down of growth is apparent after the first year. While physical growth is still rapid, mental growth is more spectacular and even more exciting to observe. Talking and questioning, using the hands, arms, and legs skillfully, curious exploring of his surroundings, growing interest in other children, all are characteristic of the child who has emerged from infancy.

The need for fitting into the cultural pattern of his family and the social group they live in makes increasing demands on the child; he is expected to learn all sorts of controls—of his voice, of noisy feet, of his crying, of his food choices, as well as of his eliminative needs. He finds he must distinguish between "mine" and "thine," and he must learn to

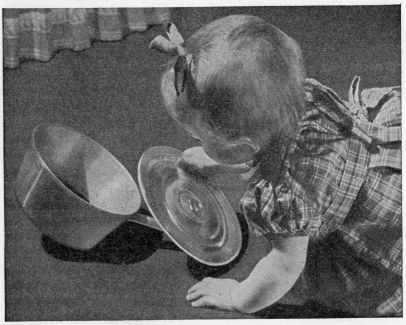

A saucepan doubles as a toy.

know what it means to share, to wait his turn, and to get along without his mother sometimes.

The pressures put upon the child will be heavy or light, depending on the degree to which his parents understand their job. Their calmness or their state of fluster and hurry-scurry will have its counterpart in the child's state of nerves. If his parents have happy, secure relationships with each other, the child will feel that too.

In such an atmosphere, children are not full of resistance and combativeness. Parents know there will be ups and downs in the children's appetites, that after the second year or so there will be days when they do not nap. Knowing that these things are natural and not something to worry about helps the mother to rest easy.

If she isn't anticipating "problems," she has more time to devote to her children's constructive needs. Play is the great avenue to a child's healthy growth of mind, body, and emotions. He need not have a wealth of toys; what he does need are creative materials, like blocks of wood, paper and paints, household odds and ends, sand, water, and suitable clothes to play in. He needs a place in which he can climb, run, dig, and romp with his companions. He should have opportunities for trips with his parents to explore the fascinating world around him.

When a child's basic needs for food, sleep, activity, companionship, and the affection of his parents are met, there will be little occasion for punishment or stern reprimands.

Little children like to have limits set that they understand. They cannot tell time, but they like the orderliness of having supper come after a bath, to be able to count on their mother's reading to them each day, to have a place for their belongings.

Parents whose children know they can count on them to listen sometimes instead of always doing all the "telling" will find less stubbornness and tantrum behavior cropping up.

If parents recognize that mistakes are to be expected but that blunders are not fatal, their children, as well as they themselves, can be more lighthearted. Of course, children sometimes feel hostile toward their parents. Parents feel hostile too. Neither need feel guilty over occasional clashes. The climate of a family is what counts, more than the occasional upsets and irritations that loom so big at the time.

Each child is an individual, and needs to be considered as one. He will grow at his own pace. We cannot influence the unfolding of his abilities any more than we can his height. What we can do is to make the setting in which he develops as free and favorable as is in our power.

THE ELEMENTARY SCHOOL YEARS

Once a child reaches school age his parents will be able to share these responsibilities with the school. But even now more of the child's "education" will go on in the home than in the school, so information about what to expect during the elementary school years is necessary to his parents.

This is a time of slower and more even growth in height and weight than in the previous years, but a time of great expansion of interests and activities. A child's friends become vastly important to him; because they influence him so much, the neighborhood a family lives in and its opportunities for wholesome play become a matter of more concern than before. Children in these years are gathering information and ideas and forming opinions about many things. The value to them of having good sound information, good models of behavior to copy, and fine ideals implanted is obvious. The movies they see and the stories they read or hear on the radio have more influence on their impressionable minds than later. In the latter part of this period, children begin to grasp abstract ideas, such as "honor," "justice," "tolerance," and "co-operation," and to form judgments about people and their actions. Parents have the challenge and the privilege of furnishing in their home life practical and concrete examples from which these ideas take shape in the child's personality and character.

Now is the time when children should be taking increased responsibility for their personal habits—dressing, bathing, eating, home study, and household tasks. Parents need to be awake to their children's growing need for independence, for a child learns to use judgment in making decisions only by having them to make.

Parents can also supplement what children learn at school by providing as much as they can of books, materials for work, and a place for creative activities. They can, by their interest, encourage children to maintain the lively interest in school work with which they start out.

The protection of their children's health is still a major concern of parents. Though the dangers of diseases are not quite so great as earlier, accidents claim a great many victims, and the need of safety education should be recognized in the home as well as in the school.

LATE CHILDHOOD AND ADOLESCENCE

After the period of more regular, comparatively even growth that characterizes middle childhood comes the time when preparation begins for new and widespread changes.

One of the main things that parents need to recognize at the pre-adolescent stage is the difference between the development of boys and girls and the great variations among individuals. Girls will be somewhat ahead of boys, on the whole, but the unevenness between two boys or two girls can be just as great. These things are of immense importance to the social adjustment of growing boys and girls; a short boy may not realize that he will in all likelihood catch up in the middle teens; a girl who gets her growth and matures early sometimes fails to realize she will not be farther advanced than others for long.

Some main factors appear over and over in children's lives, in varying proportions. To begin with, there is the economic factor. Has the child clothes like his friends or must he feel noticeably different? Does he have an allowance or ways to earn money for movies and other forms of recreation?

Then there is the personality factor. Is the child acceptable to his companions? Why do the people who like him enjoy his company? Why can't he make some of the friendships he'd like? Why is he not more comfortable in social groups?

Family attitudes and pressures are another factor for concern. Are there strains, a hard-to-dispel gloom that the child seldom gets out from under? Is mother, or father, demanding, overanxious, hovering? Or is the atmosphere one in which the boy or girl feels elated by being respected, given increasing freedom and independence, enjoyed, and allowed to grow up?

Last, there is the factor of competence and accomplishment. The child's mental and physical abilities or disabilities count much for or against his feeling that he has a place and a contribution to make. A strong boy, who is good at physical feats, is rated high. If a child lacks this physical superiority, he must make it up in some other way—by bubbling good humor, high enthusiasm, or more than ordinary friendliness. The same applies for the girl, with appearance taking the part played by physical strength or agility in the boy.

Happiness or unhappiness in school work is not always associated with actual mental ability. Schools are rare that are flexible enough to meet the great individual differences among children's strengths and weaknesses, likes and dislikes. Parents should try to avoid laying stress on marks alone; their children's efforts and the methods by which they are learning to work with and enjoy others is as yet less measurable than progress in arithmetic or spelling, but it may be of greater value as a part of their learning for life situations.

The school and teen-age years should see gradual and marked gains in ability to control emotional behavior, to take personal responsibility, and to be freed from the close parental guidance necessary in the earlier years. The adolescent lives in a world of his own. Parents cannot reënter that world, but they can stand ready to back up their children when they need backing, and to sympathize with, rather than condemn, the fumbling by which the development of mature judgment must be achieved.

THE SICK CHILD

Although somewhat detailed instructions as to the care of sick children are given in Children's Bureau Publications Nos. 8, 30, and 324, the following general suggestions should prove helpful to the home nurse.

Because children often see a doctor or nurse under unpleasant circumstances, either when they are in pain or must have inoculations, they all too frequently build up fear, and dread going to a doctor's office even for routine checkups. Much can be done to prevent such attitudes, and needs to be done, for a child's fear can hamper the doctor

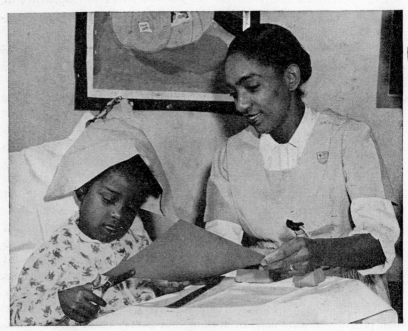

Interesting activities speed convalescence.

seriously when illness strikes. One of the good arguments for monthly, quarterly, or semiannual physical checkups, according to a child's age, while he is well is that by this means a child becomes familiar with the doctor and his office without attaching unpleasant associations to them.

It should be unnecessary to say that a child should never be threatened with the doctor, but parents have been known to say, "If you aren't good, the doctor will come and get you!"

When a child must go to a hospital, his parents should explain to him some of the things that are involved. Because fear so often attaches to the unknown, it will help him to hear about what a hospital is like and how the doctors, nurses, and other workers carry out their jobs. A child who is told in advance how his meals will be brought in on a tray, how his bed will be made with him right in it, how (if he is going to have his tonsils out, for instance) he will ride down the hall and maybe up in an elevator on a stretcher with wheels will feel less anxious when he is finally left alone in this strange new place.

When a child enters the hospital, his father or mother should be allowed to stay with him until the newness wears off. Hospital surroundings are forbidding and the strangeness frightening. A young child may suffer deeply and lastingly from the experience if all possible measures are not taken to help him feel secure and relaxed.

This does not mean, of course, that in the effort to be reassuring parents should tell a child an untruth. To say, "The doctor won't hurt you," is unfair both to the child and to the physician. It is better to say something like, "This is going to hurt, but it will be over soon. I'll hold your hand."

In some hospitals, rules about times when parents may visit are rigid. Being homesick and having to wait for days between the times he sees his father and mother may hold back a child's recovery. In other hospitals, parents are encouraged to visit at any time, and mothers may help in giving baths, serving food, reading aloud in the wards—in fact, in almost numberless ways.

Once a child is convalescing, whether in the hospital or at home, a mother's or nurse's ingenuity will be tested to find interesting but quiet occupations. Now is the time to bring out toys put away after Christmas, to ransack cupboards and drawers for odds and ends with which the child will enjoy making things, and to bring out the mail-order catalog and old magazines. An older child may like to learn to knit or crochet, or to make a scrapbook of family snapshots that have been accumulating.

The use of the radio will need to be rather carefully watched, so that the convalescent may not be emotionally keyed up by programs that are overexciting or fear-producing. To have a wide selection of books from the public library for the child who is old enough to read will be worth the effort, for then he can make choices according to his needs and interests at the moment.

Medical Supervision

If a child is being seen regularly by a doctor, the doctor will probably notice any slowly developing signs of disease before the child becomes sick. The sudden changes that usher in acute illnesses, however, are more likely to be noticed first by a child's mother.

Signs of fatigue, such as refusal to eat a meal, fussiness, or irritability, should disappear after a good night's sleep. But the child who habitually has little appetite for food, who is cranky, pale, tired, and underweight, is often a sick child. Sometimes these symptoms are the outcome of poor habit training, but more often they are not. It is especially important for any child who is constantly below par to be under a doctor's regular supervision.

As in adults, a good deal of sickness may be prevented in children by:

1. Regular visits to the doctor.
2. Maintaining immunization up to date (*see* Chart of Selected Communicable Diseases).
3. Keeping children away from those who are sick.
4. Teaching good health habits.

When children are sick, call the doctor early, put them to bed, keep them away from others, feed them lightly, and keep them warm and quiet.

Symptoms of Illness

By observing a baby or young child carefully, one soon learns to recognize any changes from the usual behavior. The chief symptoms of sickness to look for in babies and young children are:

1. Loss of appetite.
2. Listlessness during the day or drowsiness or restlessness, especially at night.
3. Irritability.
4. Fever.
5. Running nose, sneezing, and coughing.
6. Diarrhea.
7. Rash.

8. Vomiting.
9. Convulsions.
10. Stiff neck.

The mother should learn how to take a rectal temperature (*see* Taking the Temperature, p. 141) and should know her baby's habits well enough to recognize any change from ordinary behavior.

Crying. A baby's cry is a language in itself. The wakeful, hungry, persistent cry before feeding time; the slightly angry, fussy cry of the baby who is uncomfortable (wet, cold, or tired); the resentful, hearty cry of the baby getting his bath or not getting what he wants—all these cries should soon be familiar to the parent's ear—so much so that the high, sharp cry of pain, the shrill, breathless crying of fright or pain, the irritable crying of fever, and the low moaning or plaintive whimper of a weak or really sick baby are easily recognized as warnings. A hoarse, choked cry is not natural either and should be investigated at once.

Restlessness. A well baby sleeps quietly and at regular intervals. A sick baby may pitch and toss, roll his head from side to side, move around in his sleep, or twitch and moan. Restlessness is usually a sign of discomfort somewhere and the experienced mother learns to watch her baby and detect such movements as rubbing an ear, bringing the knees up if the pain is in the abdomen or stomach, or pulling the head backward. Make a note of the baby's discomfort. Take his temperature, and if there is a fever, rigidity over the abdomen, or the neck seems stiff, report the symptoms to the doctor.

A baby will be restless on hot nights just as adults are; sponging with cool water and a change of position may quiet him.

Fever. Children have fevers for slight causes, and yet a slight fever that persists may be serious. When a baby or child has a fever:

1. Put him to bed in a room by himself if possible.
2. Notify the doctor.
3. Give a light diet in the case of a child; for the baby withdraw all food except milk and water.

Rash. By the time the rash of a communicable disease appears, except in the case of chickenpox, the child is usually sick enough to have warranted a doctor's visit. The most infectious period of the communicable disease *precedes* the appearance of the rash; the rash simply confirms the doctor's diagnosis. The other symptoms of communicable disease (*see* Chart of Selected Communicable Diseases, p. 218) are therefore also im-

portant for the mother to note. Rashes may likewise be caused by food
or other allergies, by improper food, or by poisons such as poison ivy.

Tell the doctor about any rash that appears on the baby's body. Tell
him where the rash is, what it looks like, and whether the child has a
fever. Prickly heat or heat rash may appear on the baby's body if he is
too warm. Take away wool and feather pillows, lighten his clothing, and
bathe the skin with lukewarm water to which baking soda (2 tablespoonfuls to 1 gallon) has been added. If a heat rash does not clear up in a few
days, the doctor should see it; the rash may be the result of food or an
infection.

Vomiting. Babies "spit up" easily and the line between spitting up and
vomiting is not easily defined. A baby who has gas, has taken too much
food, has taken it too fast, or has been jolted about after feeding will spit
up; excitement and fatigue may cause it. It usually occurs soon after
feeding and the material looks much as it did when it went down. Vomiting is a deeper action; the stomach empties itself more completely, and
the material may be more digested and may be odorous. Slower, quieter,
smaller feedings, with a pause midway to "bubble" the baby (*see* p. 200)
and rest afterward, may correct spitting up. The doctor should be told if
the practice continues and if vomiting occurs more than once without
apparent reason.

Diarrhea. Diarrhea has many causes. A safe course is to restrict food
temporarily and call the doctor if the symptoms persist. Boiled water may
be given. Boil the diapers. Keep other children away. Be careful to wash
the hands after handling the baby and his belongings; if there is fever
with the diarrhea, stop *all* feeding and report the symptoms to the doctor. If there is a delay of more than 12 hours in getting a doctor or a
doctor's advice, give half of the baby's formula, diluted with boiled
water, or continue breast-feeding if breast-fed.

Nursing Care

Most of the principles of home nursing care described in this book are
applicable to children and the same routines in carrying out procedures
are followed—adjusted, of course, to the size of the child. Any adaptations or changes in materials for children are noted in the list of procedures.

As far as possible, the child's normal daily schedule should be followed. This makes it easier to return to good habits of eating, sleeping,
and elimination when the child recovers. A sick child needs plenty of

sleep. Plan regular nap times; darken the room; maintain quiet; and see that the air is fresh but *not* cold.

It is just as important to keep a careful record of the home care given a sick child as to keep one for an adult. Symptoms and reactions in children develop fast and disappear fast; their seriousness cannot be judged by their duration or their effect on the child. Report everything unusual in the sick child's behavior. It may have significance to the doctor.

THE HANDICAPPED CHILD

The problem of the handicapped child—the child who must remain in bed for weeks and may even have to learn to live with a lifetime handicap—is a special one and as a rule needs skillful handling. The child must not be coddled; yet he must learn to live within the limit of his strength. He must not be overprotected so that he develops fears or inhibitions; yet his way must be made safe and adjusted to his need. Certain rough games will be out of the question. Often advice may be sought from a child psychologist, or the child may do better in a convalescent home among others of his age similarly afflicted. Circumstances alter cases and parents should seek the best advice possible, especially if they see their child becoming irritable, shy, depressed, or fearful of meeting the problems of everyday life.

Visiting teachers are available in many communities for bedridden children of school age. Special classes for the handicapped may be the answer for children able to be up and about, while for some serious conditions special institutional care is the best solution of the problem. There are a number of institutions providing such care, in addition to services for acute illness available in children's hospitals—for example, homes for crippled children, cardiac patients, the deaf, blind, and others. Ask the doctor or the local or state health department for further information. (*See also* The Convalescent Patient, p. 70, *and* Rehabilitation, p. 82.)

MAINTAINING GOOD HEALTH

When all the bodily functions are working together smoothly and naturally so that the demands of life can be met capably and calmly, we say a person is healthy.

Health is never just physical. Our feelings or emotions are affected by the condition of the body as well. Thus, when a person has a headache, he is usually cross and uninterested in work and finds it hard to concentrate. When the mind is ill, there are nearly always physical symptoms such as sleeplessness, headache, and fatigue.

Most of us come into the world with a perfect body. Whether it will meet the demands made upon it depends largely upon the intelligent care and training we receive when young and upon the way we treat our bodies after we are old enough to be responsible for our actions. There are outward signs which we usually associate with physical health, such as a good appetite, restful sleep at night, regular bowel and bladder movements, clear eyes and skin, uncoated tongue, sweet breath, glossy hair, upright posture, a contented facial expression, and abundant energy.

A person in good physical health is usually quite unaware of his body's mechanism; it functions smoothly, takes him to the places he wants to go, responds to his demands, and is refreshed and ready to start again after securing food and sleep. There are also outward signs of mental health. We think of a well-adjusted person as one who is happy in his work and play, interested in his friends and all that goes on around him, likes and is liked by others, and has no recurrent nervous habits, peculiar moods, or repeated spells of temper.

But the *outward* signs of health are far from being the whole story. The doctor looks much deeper for the evidences of physical and mental health or illness. He studies the temperature of the body, the pulse rate, the blood pressure, the sounds made by the heart and lungs as they perform their function, the chemistry of the blood, and the process of digestion. Many other tests and measurements go into a complete physical examination; indeed, so many are needed to determine the presence or absence of illness or unusual physical or emotional changes that only a doctor should ever attempt to make a judgment. Similarly, the doctor must decide through further testing whether a person is mentally well or ill and what kind of mental illness is present.

Medical Supervision

One of the simplest ways to be reasonably sure that the body and mind are functioning well is to have a routine, complete medical examination at regular intervals. Authorities suggest an annual examination but the age and condition of the individual will determine the interval between examinations. For example, preschool children should be seen by the family doctor or a pediatrician (children's doctor) at least every 6 months; an adult who has recovered from a serious illness may have to see a doctor every 2 or 3 weeks. Persons over 40 should make an annual health examination a routine practice.

The principle of a regular checkup of the body applies also to the care of the teeth and eyes. The dentist and eye doctor will suggest the schedule best suited to the individual's needs.

Aside from the comfort and assurance a routine health checkup brings, it actually pays in the long run because small defects or undesirable changes in the body can be found before they become major problems requiring expensive repairs and loss of time from work. The examinations also give the doctor the chance to offer the best and most up-to-date protection from communicable disease (*see* Chart of Selected Communicable Diseases, p. 218) and the most recent and effective treatments, appliances, or aids for whatever condition one may have. Hardly a year passes without the discovery of some improvement in ways to care for the human body and mind. It is sensible and pays to take advantage of these discoveries and to give oneself the same thorough overhauling that one periodically gives a car or any other piece of delicate machinery.

Good health habits play a part in maintaining good health, and their importance is appreciated when the functions of the body are understood. It is suggested that Red Cross classes in home nursing, which include instruction in recognizing symptoms of illness and its causes, can be helpful in maintaining personal and family health. It is especially important that every individual learn to recognize the symptoms of communicable diseases and of such killers as cancer, heart disease, and tuberculosis, as these may develop at any age.

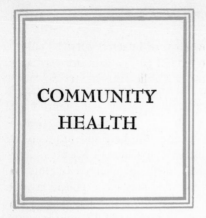

COMMUNITY HEALTH

8

A COMMUNITY has a legal and moral responsibility to protect the health and well-being of its citizens, whether they live in a city, a village, or out in the country. The home nurse has a responsibility to herself and to her family to know and make use of the health resources available in her community. She should consider her functions within the home as being in harmony with and actually contributing to the protection of the health of the entire community.

Community health protection is known as "public health" and is defined as the science and art of preventing disease, prolonging life, and promoting mental and physical health and efficiency. Experience has shown that, to achieve these goals, there must be organized efforts to keep our surroundings in a clean, sanitary, and safe condition, control community infections, educate the individual in principles of personal health, supply medical and nursing services for preventive treatment and early diagnosis of disease, and develop social machinery that will insure to every individual a standard of living adequate for the maintenance of health. Four essentials needed for a successful community health program are trained workers, adequate funds, proper health regulations, and favorable public opinion.

Under the American system of government, the care of the public health is regarded as primarily the responsibility of the health departments of the individual states and political subdivisions—the city, the county, and sometimes the township. However, some states have insufficient funds to provide a satisfactory health program without federal aid. They may have unusual disease problems, such as malaria, hookworm, Rocky Mountain spotted fever, or certain occupational diseases, and therefore may need the assistance of available federal experts with special training to combat these problems.

The federal government also studies national and international health problems and helps protect the country from the introduction of diseases from outside the country. It helps control the transmission of disease from state to state by regulating the movement of infected persons, animals, and goods. Health activities of the federal government are carried on chiefly by or under the supervision of the Public Health Service, the Children's Bureau of the Federal Security Agency, and the U.S. Department of Agriculture.

In addition to the official or governmental agencies engaged in public health work in a community, there are usually one or more nonofficial or so-called voluntary agencies that supplement the work of the health department. These agencies are supported wholly or in part by private funds. A tuberculosis association financed through the sale of Christmas seals or a visiting nurse association supported by fees from patients and contributions from the local Community Chest are illustrations of such agencies. Citizens groups acting either in an advisory or administrative capacity help keep the services of such agencies close to the needs of the people they serve. On the national level, such voluntary organizations as the American Public Health Association, the National Organization for Public Health Nursing, the American Cancer Society, the National Foundation for Infantile Paralysis, and the American National Red Cross have contributed much to the progress made in public health. Most of these organizations have state or local subdivisions.

All these agencies, tax-supported or voluntary, exist for the benefit of the individual and the community. There is hardly a question regarding public health that cannot be answered by their experts. Many of these agencies will send health education material upon request, as well as answer questions.

THE HEALTH DEPARTMENT

The health department, which is tax supported, is the authorized agency created by a city, town, county, or state to preserve and protect the public health.

The majority of local health departments are located in the municipal or county building near other county and city departments, such as education, welfare, engineering, and public works. This is also usually the building in which births and deaths are registered. One should know where the health department is located and what health services are available. Not all health departments offer the same services, this depends somewhat upon the particular health needs of the community and the public's willingness to support the department, but in general the responsibilities of the local health department in a city cover the fields here listed. Services in rural areas are usually more limited.

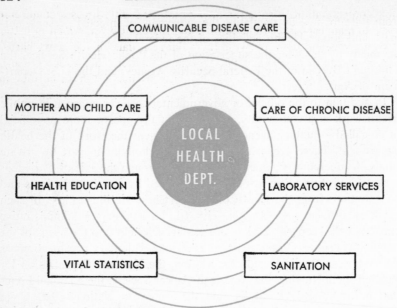

Usual functions of a local health department.

Protection of the Water Supply

The water supply of a community should be pure and sufficient to meet the community's needs. There should be adequate means for storage in reservoirs and for purification as well as for protection against pollution by sewage, which may harbor the germs of typhoid or other diseases. Meeting these essentials requires accurate engineering knowledge and the skill of an expert trained and experienced in sanitation.

Anyone having any question regarding the safety of the home water supply should consult the health department. For those living in a rural area, pamphlets prepared for distribution or an inspector from this department may help decide where to locate a well in relation to the farm buildings and how to protect it from contamination. Occasionally a flood, broken water main, or other emergency will interrupt or contaminate the water supply. When this happens, obey the warnings of the health department and boil the drinking water. Serious illness may be avoided by following directions exactly at such times.

Protection of the Milk Supply

The milk supply of communities must be protected to safeguard human lives. If disease germs are present in the milk, they multiply rapidly if the milk is warm. Human handling of milk exposes it to pos-

sible contamination. Also, cows may be infected with diseases communicable to man, especially tuberculosis, and undulant fever, which in cattle
is contagious abortion. To avoid these dangers, dairy herds, dairy barns,
plants distributing milk and milk products (butter, cheese, ice cream),
and employees must be inspected regularly by the health authorities to
assure that sanitary standards are being maintained. Sterilization of
bottles and other utensils, safe collection and pasteurization, and adequate refrigeration of milk are necessary to insure protection from
contamination.

In small or rural communities or where no supervision is available,
every housewife must take precautions to protect her family from milk-
borne diseases. If possible, obtain milk from dairies or farmers whose
cattle are tested for tuberculosis. If milk is not pasteurized at its source
—that is, heated to destroy bacteria—it should be either boiled or pasteurized at home.

To pasteurize milk at home, the homemaker may use an approved
home pasteurizer (there are several commercial ones on the market) or
either of the following methods:

1. After the water in the bottom of a double boiler has been brought
to a vigorous boil, place the inner container with the milk in it in the
outer container; cover it; and continue to apply the same heat for 10
minutes.

2. Heat the milk in an open saucepan over a hot flame to 165° F.,
using a dairy or candy thermometer, and stir constantly. Then immediately place the vessel in cold water and continue stirring until the milk
is cool, changing the water when it warms up. If a dependable thermometer is not available, bring the milk to a boil instead.

Method *1* produces a cooked flavor, which may be objected to, but
is considered a safer method than *2*.[1]

Evaporated milk and dried milk may be cheaper and safer than fresh
milk in many communities, especially if there is a question as to the
safety of the fresh milk.

Protection of the Food Supply

The community should provide adequate safeguards for its food supply. All bakeries, groceries, markets, shops, stores, and storage houses
should be supervised and required to protect food according to prevail-
ing sanitary regulations. All food should be kept clean and should be

---

[1] Adapted by permission from Public Health Reports, Vol. 65, No. 6, Feb. 10,
1950.

protected from dust, vermin, and flies and other insects, as well as from careless handling by persons who may transfer disease through food. Definite illnesses have been traced, for example, to a cook's infected finger. Food served to the public at special functions, such as church suppers or auctions, may be the source of an epidemic of food poisoning unless the same precautions are taken as are required for public eating places. Food factories and places concerned with the preparation, storage, or sale of meat, poultry, game, or fish—including shellfish such as oysters and clams—are subject to inspection and are usually allowed to operate only under a license obtained from the health department.

Prevention and Control of Communicable Diseases

General measures of prevention include such items as informing people about communicable diseases and their control; immunization of people against specific diseases, when possible; enforcement of health laws and regulations to prevent the spread of communicable disease from a sick person to others who may be susceptible; location and control of carriers of various diseases; examination of animals which may spread disease and taking proper measures for its control, for example, detention of dogs that may have rabies and disposition of cattle with tuberculosis; and attention to general sanitary measures such as rat control and destroying breeding places of flies and mosquitoes.

Some health departments supply nursing service on a visit basis for instruction and care in communicable disease in the home. In some localities this service is available from the Visiting Nurse Association.

Control of Noncommunicable Diseases

The prevalence of some noncommunicable diseases has become a matter of concern to all, since many people may be affected and the costs, both to the community and to the individual, may be high. Health departments in many communities have joined with various private agencies to inform the public of potential dangers, to offer diagnostic services, and when possible to take steps for the prevention and care of these diseases. Examples of such activities are cancer control programs, or the eradication of ragweed, one of the common causes of hay fever, asthma, and other allergic conditions.

Health Records

The health department keeps a record of all births and deaths (vital statistics) occurring in the community. This department will issue duplicate copies of birth certificates to individuals who may wish to establish their identity.

Clinic Services

It is customary for the health department to conduct one or more clinics for health services. These may be purely in the preventive field—diagnostic clinics and health examination clinics such as well-baby conferences—or the health department may supply treatments to those unable to pay for the service of private physicians. Examples of the latter are clinics for the diagnosis and treatment of venereal disease and tuberculosis, and for immunization against diphtheria, whooping cough, and smallpox.

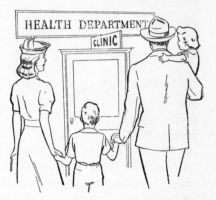

Detailed information concerning clinic services may be obtained by visiting, writing, or telephoning the health department.

Utilize the services of the local health department.

Nursing Service

Nearly all health departments employ one or more public health nurses. They may visit homes where there is a health problem, serve in clinics, teach classes in mother and baby care, give care to the sick in the home, and assist the health officer in many phases of the health program. Public health nurses are professional registered nurses with special training in public health in addition to their school of nursing preparation. They may be called on for advice on health problems or for information on where to go for help.

Health Education

The health department assumes considerable responsibility for informing the public how to maintain health and avoid disease. Frequently there is someone in the department assigned especially to answer questions, to provide health leaflets, and to plan radio and newspaper publicity. In times of emergency, such as epidemics, or when a special campaign is launched to inform the public regarding some new health service, direct messages may be expected from the health department. The health department is the bureau of information regarding health services in the

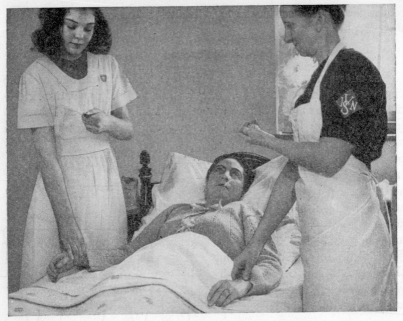

Visiting nurse guides the home nurse.

community. It can serve more effectively when each member of the community understands its functions and works coöperatively with it in the control of disease and promotion of health.

Industrial Health and Safety

A plan for the health and safety of industrial workers is recognized as an important part in a health program. Many state health departments and several local health departments have established programs in cooperation with private industry for the prevention of occupational diseases and other hazards.

School Health Service

Providing full- or part-time school physicians and nurses in schools may be a responsibility of the health department or it may be one of the board of education. Private schools, including parochial schools, may provide their own health service. Each community has a right to expect, however, that its children be protected, in so far as possible, from communicable disease while at school, that their physical condition is routinely checked, and that they are learning sound and safe health habits during school hours.

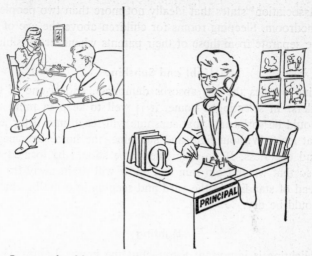

Parents should notify school authorities when child is ill.

HOUSING

The Public Health Service of the Federal Security Agency has listed the essentials of a healthful home environment as:

1. Space enough for ordinary family needs.
2. Absence of excessive dampness.
3. Sufficient ventilation, heat, and light.
4. Adequate play space and sunshine for children.
5. A pure and sufficient water supply.
6. Sanitary refuse and sewage disposal.
7. Screening against flies and mosquitoes.
8. Protection against other insects and rodents.
9. Protection against fire hazards and other accident risks.

Space Requirements

It is not necessary to have a separate house to live in, although it is highly desirable for many reasons. An individual house usually provides yard space for the children, room for a vegetable garden, light, sunshine, and free circulation of air. These conditions are seldom available to the city dweller living in an apartment or flat. In any type of home it is important to avoid overcrowding—too many people sharing limited space—and to see that there are the necessary sanitary conveniences.

A subcommittee on the hygiene of housing of the American Public

Health Association[2] states that ideally not more than two people should share a bedroom. Sleeping rooms for children above the age of 2 years should be separate from those of their parents whenever possible.

Light and Sunshine

Sunshine purifies the air, absorbs dampness, and is one of the best germ killers. In selecting a home, it is well to keep in mind that the house should be so located that sunshine will reach into it for a part of the day at least. Without light and sunshine, the home becomes damp, chilly, and cheerless. If possible, the home should be located on high ground, so that water from rain and snow will drain away from buildings instead of standing in the yard and seeping into the basement. The cellar should be dry.

Lighting

Good lighting is important throughout the house. Lamps with light-colored, but not transparent, shades should be provided in sufficient numbers to meet the needs of every member of the family. Inexpensive reading lamps can be purchased equipped with a device to soften the light and reduce glare. This is called semi-indirect lighting and is much less trying on the eyes than is direct light. The kitchen should be one of the lightest and cheeriest of the rooms in the house, because the preparation of food may involve much time and close eyework.

The homemaker should check the places in the house most in need of lighting, day or night, to prevent accidents. These points are usually the front and back doorsteps, the cellar stairs, uneven floor levels from room to room, and the stair landings. If there is a member of the household or a guest who is likely to be up in the night, he should be familiar with the light switches or be provided with a light.

Heating and Ventilation

Heating and ventilation are chiefly winter problems, although modern heating systems that also provide for air conditioning add a great deal to summer comfort. Too much heat in the home causes the body to give off more moisture in perspiration and makes it more sensitive to drafts and chilling. Too little heat often makes the body less resistant to colds and tends to prevent normal elimination through the skin. A room temperature between 65° and 75° is satisfactory to most people doing active

[2] Subcommittee on the Hygiene of Housing of the Committee on Research and Standards of the American Public Health Association.

work. Elderly people, invalids, and those who are less active usually require more heat because the blood circulates less rapidly and the body produces less heat of its own. It is desirable to have wall thermometers strategically placed throughout the house for convenience in checking the temperature. Sleeping rooms can be kept somewhat cooler than living rooms.

Home Water Supply

If one lives in a city or large town he can be reasonably certain that it will have a safe water supply as long as the plumbing pipes are kept in good condition so that there is no possibility of leakage from sewer pipes getting into the water used for household purposes.

If one must depend upon a well or cistern for the water supply, he should know the conditions that make it safe and those that might be questioned. Detailed instructions for the construction and protection of wells and cisterns may be obtained through the local health department.

If there is any doubt about the safety of water, it should be boiled for 3 minutes; this treatment will kill disease germs, but it tends to remove oxygen and makes the water taste flat. Water used for brushing teeth, washing dishes, or cleaning vegetables should be as pure and free from bacteria as drinking water.

Sewage and Refuse Disposal

In cities and large towns the sewer carries away the liquid waste from the community to a place where it may be disposed of in a sanitary manner without endangering the health of the people.

Small communities sometimes depend upon individual cesspools, which are deep pits or tanks into which all wastes from the home are discharged by means of pipes and running water. While it is possible to keep the cesspool drainage from getting into the water supply, there is always danger that this may happen. The modern method of sewage disposal for individual country homes is the septic tank. This is a large tank located underground at least 50 feet from a well or water pipes. The solid matter settles to the bottom of the tank or floats on the surface of the water until it has been changed into liquid form by the action of bacteria. The tank has an outlet through which the liquid part of the sewage is drained into pipes that carry it to a nearby field, where it is discharged into the top soil (the upper 20 to 24 inches of ground). Here, again, bacteria act upon it, changing it into food for plants and making it harmless.

In communities without a modern sewer system and in a large percentage of rural homes, the outdoor privy is still in use. A privy can be made safe, but unless it is properly placed and constructed there is great danger that drainage from it may reach the well or cistern and pollute the water supply. There is also danger that flies may carry disease germs from the privy to the house and so contaminate food and eating utensils.

Information regarding construction of cesspools, septic tanks, or outdoor privies may be obtained from local or state health departments or directly from the Public Health Service, Federal Security Agency, Washington 25, D. C.

Flies and Mosquitoes

Flies breed and feed on the body discharges of men and animals and on all kinds of decaying vegetable matter. Barnyards and the back alleys of cities and towns are favorite places for them to live. Since we know that flies carry disease germs, it is obvious that everything possible must be done to protect the home against them. The best way to do this is to prevent the accumulation of the material in which they breed. This is the reason cities require that garbage be kept in covered cans and removed and destroyed regularly and that alleys be kept clean.

The next step in protecting the home against flies is the screening of all windows and doors. These should fit tightly and be kept in good condition if they are to be of any value. Screens should be fine enough to keep out mosquitoes and other small insects as well as flies. Sixteen-mesh wire is advised by the U. S. Department of Agriculture.

Mosquito control is as important as fly control, because certain kinds of mosquitoes carry disease. Any standing water affords a good breeding place for mosquitoes. The householder can help control mosquitoes by preventing the accumulation of stagnant water in such places as tin cans, rain barrels, open drains, puddles, and pools. Instructions for mosquito control can be obtained through the local department of health or the U. S. Department of Agriculture. DDT and other insecticides, when properly applied, are also effective in controlling flies and mosquitoes in and around the house.

Rats

Places around the home where rats can breed and multiply should be eliminated, and rubbish and garbage that may attract them should not be allowed to accumulate. All holes or places of entry to the house should be blocked in such a way that the rats cannot gnaw through them. Traps, if used in sufficient numbers, may help to control rats, but great care must be taken to set traps where children or domestic animals cannot get into them.

Poisons should always be used under the guidance of an expert to prevent accidents. Poison bait is dangerous because it is sometimes picked up by children or pets; also, poisoned rats may die in the walls or under the house and cause a disagreeable odor.

Fire Prevention

The ideal home is fireproof or at least fire-resistant. Modern apartment houses and the new materials for individual homes stress this safety feature. In individual homes there should be at least one small fire extinguisher kept in the kitchen. However, it is preferable to have one on each floor. Everyone should know how to call the fire department, if there is one available. Fire escapes should be kept clear of obstructions.

Danger of fire arises from overheated stoves; candles or unscreened fires; defective lighting, heating, or wiring; defective electrical appliances; clogged chimney flues; accumulation of rubbish in cellars, attics, or on stairways; and careless use of matches and flammable materials such as kerosene and cleaning fluids.

To safeguard against fire, it is advisable to clear out rubbish, keep matches in a safe place out of the reach of children, screen open fires, keep curtains away from any flame, check all electrical connections and stoves regularly and repair any defect promptly, keep chimneys clean, refrain from smoking in bed, use care when handling lighted candles, and use flammable materials according to directions.

Prevention of Accidents

There are other accident hazards in the home besides that of fire. The hazards may be reduced in the following ways:

1. Anchor loose rugs on slippery floors by using rubber or cork mats under them or by stitching rubber rings, such as those used on preserve jars, along the edges. Avoid placing loose rugs at the top or bottom of stairs.

2. Keep stairways, landings, and cellars well lighted. Paint the bottom and top steps white. Guard against slipping on the stairs. Provide handrails.

3. Use stepladders instead of chairs to reach high places.

4. Keep knives, razors, scissors, or other cutting tools in a safe place and out of reach of children.

5. Keep medicine separate from cleaning fluids, paints, weed poisons, or other dangerous compounds and out of reach of children.

6. See that small children are not alone in the kitchen when food is cooking, water is heating, the washing machine is running, or if gas taps are within their reach.

7. Prevent boiling over of liquid on a gas stove, which may put out the flame and allow the gas to escape.

8. Never run a car in a closed garage because of the danger from carbon monoxide poisoning.

9. Be careful in the use of electrical appliances. Disconnect an electric iron when finished with its use, and avoid touching an electric light or other connection when standing on a wet floor or in the bathtub.

10. Provide handrails on the stairs or gate protection at the head of the stairs for children; handrails in the bathtub are especially advised for elderly people.

11. Use care when handling explosives such as gasoline or cleaning fluids.

12. Be sure guns are emptied of ammunition or kept out of the reach of children.

RECREATION

Allowing time for recreation is an important factor contributing to the health of the individual. Many communities provide playgrounds, centers, and other recreational facilities for persons of all ages, which supplement the recreational facilities of the home. The home nurse can contribute to the health and well-being of her family by taking an active interest in the building and maintenance of safe, clean, and healthful recreational facilities and by encouraging family members to participate in these ventures.

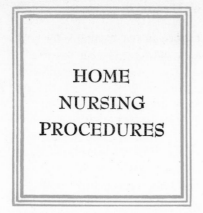

HOME NURSING PROCEDURES

9

GENERAL INFORMATION

SIMPLE nursing procedures that can be carried out in the home are presented here step by step. It is difficult to visualize some of these without a demonstration or to acquire skill without guided practice. For this reason, it is expected that those who are responsible for giving this care in the home will have completed the Red Cross Home Nursing courses, or received help from a public health or other professional nurse, and that this section of the book will serve as a handy reference.

The home nurse should remember, however, that there is an art as well as a technic involved in giving good nursing care and that she is caring for a *person* and not just a *patient*. The development of a healthy mental attitude may be as important to the recovery of the patient as the required physical care.

It is taken for granted that the home nurse has the doctor's assurance that a patient's condition is such that he can be cared for safely in the home. For patients who do not need highly skilled care or special hospital equipment, the warm, friendly atmosphere of the home is often more conducive to recovery than the more formal, impersonal environment of the hospital.

When caring for a patient at home, whether he is confined to bed or not, the home nurse will find it helpful to remember the following things:

1. It is easier to care for the patient and do the other necessary household tasks if a schedule is planned for the day.
2. It will save time if:
   a. Everything needed is collected before care is given, and things are cleared away and cleansed promptly afterward. When the same treatment is given frequently, the necessary articles should be kept together on a tray.
   b. Unnecessary laundry can be avoided by protecting the bedding.
   c. Work on one side of the bed should be completed, when possible, before going to the other side.

d. Menus should be planned in advance, and food suitable for both the family and patient should be prepared whenever possible.

3. The home nurse will help safeguard her own health or conserve her strength if she:

a. Washes her hands before and after giving care to a patient.

b. Wears comfortable, low-heeled shoes to lessen back strain and short-sleeved, washable clothing to permit freedom of action.

c. Maintains good working posture.

d. Gets someone to help lift a heavy or helpless patient.

e. Obtains the patient's help. When lifting, turning, or moving a patient in bed, the home nurse should ask or help the patient to bend his knees so that he can be moved with less effort. The home nurse and the patient should act upon an agreed signal. For example, when helping the patient lift his hips, both will act on the count of three.

f. Avoids direct contact with nose and throat spray when working in close contact with the patient.

4. The home nurse will help keep her patient as comfortable as possible and also help his recovery if she:

a. Protects him from further infection by preventing exposure to the nose and throat spray or soiled hands of the home nurse or visitors.

b. Checks to see that the room is warm and that the patient is protected against drafts when giving him a bath or treatment.

c. Explains what is to be done and, if he is able, how he may help.

d. Helps the patient maintain good bed posture at all times. When giving a treatment, she should make sure the patient is in the correct position to receive care and that he is comfortable, warm, and dry during and after the treatment. A lightweight, washable blanket is often more convenient to use during baths or treatments than the usual top bedclothes and may save laundry.

e. Maintains a cheerful, wholesome mental attitude at all times to build the patient's morale and confidence.

PUTTING ON AND TAKING OFF A COVER-ALL APRON

Purpose. To provide a means of helping prevent the spread of disease from the patient or to the patient.

The home nurse should wear some type of cover-all apron when entering the sickroom to give care to the patient and take it off when leaving the room, hanging it near the door of the sickroom in readiness for use.

Procedure

1. Don the apron.
   a. Slip the arms into the sleeves of the apron without touching the outside, which will be next to the patient.
   b. Fasten at the neck and waist for ease in working.
2. Wash the hands after caring for the patient.
3. Remove the apron.
   a. Unfasten.
   b. Slip the arms out of the sleeves.
   c. Hang—keep inside in and clean.

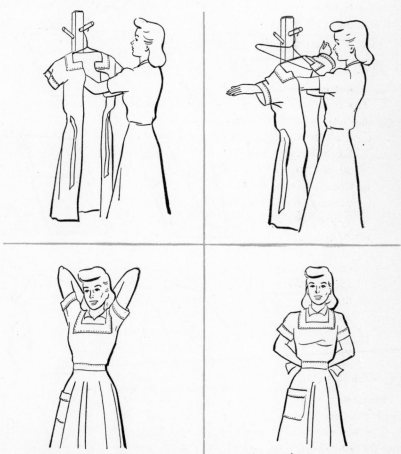

Use a cover-all apron when caring for the sick in the home.

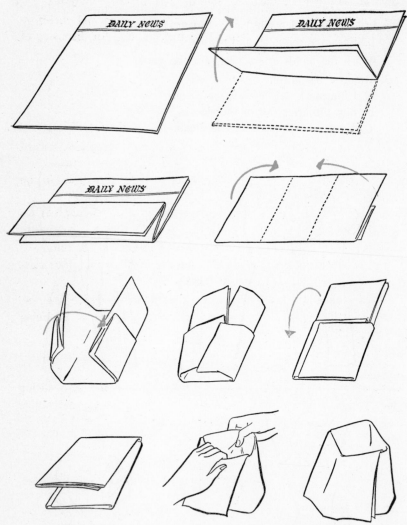

Steps in making a newspaper bag for waste disposal.

MAKING A NEWSPAPER BAG

Purpose. To provide a means of safe disposal of waste material.

Waste material from a sickroom may carry infection and therefore must be disposed of properly. Paper bags may be used for disposing of many types of waste.

Equipment
Double sheet of newspaper

Procedure

1. Place the newspaper, folded in half, with the center fold toward the person making the bag.

2. Bring the top edge of the upper sheet of the paper down to the center fold. This makes a cuff.

3. Turn the paper over, smooth side up, keeping the center fold toward the person throughout the procedure.

4. Fold it in thirds from the sides; crease well to hold the fold.

5. Lock by tucking one whole side under the cuff of the other side.

6. Bring the flap over the locked cuff.

7. Place a hand in the opening at the top; stand the bag up; shape.

8. Use the flap as a cover for the bag or as a means of fastening the bag to the side of the bed.

WASHING THE HANDS

Purpose. The home nurse washes her hands before and after caring for the patient to help protect the patient, the home nurse, and others from infection.

Equipment

Basin or bowl
Running water or container of clean warm water
Clean towels
Waste container for soiled towels

Soap
Waste pail or other means of disposing of liquid waste

Roll up the sleeves if wearing long ones. Remove the wrist watch, or push it up on the arm. Remove jewelry that is likely to hurt the patient or collect lint and other soil.

The hands should be washed under running water; where this is not available, pour water from the container.

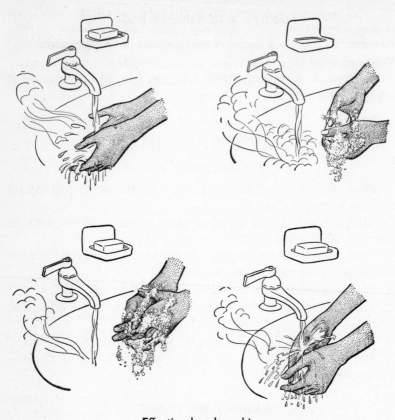

Effective hand washing.

Procedure

1. Keep the hands lowered over the basin throughout the entire procedure.

2. Wet the hands so that the soap will lather.

3. Soap hands well, working up a lather.

4. Rinse the soap (if using a bar), leaving it clean for the next use.

5. Use friction, rubbing well between the fingers and around the nails, and be sure to wash the entire hand and wrist.

6. Rinse the hands to allow the first dirt to run off.

7. Soap again, being sure to work up a good lather, and using friction as before between the fingers and around the nails.

8. Rinse the soap.

9. Rinse the hands again, getting all the dirt off this time.

10. Dry the hands well. Wet skin or dried soap on the skin may cause chapping, and breaks in the skin may admit infection. Also, chapped hands are unsightly and are uncomfortable for both the patient and the nurse.

11. Discard the towels in a waste container.

12. Dispose of the waste container.

Essential Points To Remember.

1. Hold the hands down over the basin and wash under clean running water.

2. Use friction.

3. Dry well.

TAKING THE TEMPERATURE

Purpose. To determine the patient's temperature in order to help the doctor make a diagnosis and prescribe treatment.

Fever or clinical thermometers differ from most other thermometers in that the mercury remains at the highest point registered until it is shaken down. They are fragile and must be handled with care, kept in a safe place when not in use, and protected from heat. The temperature is usually taken by the mouth or rectum, but may also be taken at the armpit. For an accurate reading, keep the thermometer in place in the body for at least 3 minutes, except when the temperature is taken at the armpit, in which case leave the thermometer in place for 10 minutes.

Some mouth thermometers have a slender bulb about ½ inch in length. Others have a short, stubby bulb. Only thermometers with stubby bulbs should be used to take rectal temperatures as there is less danger of their breaking and injuring the patient. If only one thermometer can

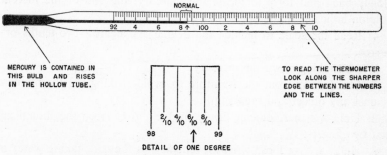

NORMAL

MERCURY IS CONTAINED IN
THIS BULB AND RISES
IN THE HOLLOW TUBE.

TO READ THE THERMOMETER
LOOK ALONG THE SHARPER
EDGE BETWEEN THE NUMBERS
AND THE LINES.

²/₁₀ ⁴/₁₀ ⁶/₁₀ ⁸/₁₀

98   99

DETAIL OF ONE DEGREE

Diagrammatic drawing of thermometer.

be purchased, it should be a thermometer with a stubby bulb, which can be used for taking temperatures by any of the above methods.

Thermometers have two parts:

1. *The bulb end:* This holds the mercury and is the part that is placed in the mouth; it must be kept clean.

2. *The glass tube:* Through this tube the mercury rises and on it are shown the lines and numbers that indicate the degrees. The column of mercury can be seen between the lines and the numbers—through a ridge which extends the length of the tube. When handling the thermometer, always grasp it by the top of the tube.

When the thermometer is in position for taking the temperature, the heat of the body expands the mercury and pushes it up into the tube.

The long lines on the tube of the thermometer are the degrees—94, 95, 96, and so on—while the short lines between are each two-tenths of a degree. However space allows room for printing only the even numbers. The normal temperature by the mouth is usually 98.6° F. (Fahrenheit), which is indicated on the tube by a small arrow.

If the home nurse cannot read the thermometer after taking a temperature, she should cleanse it according to the directions given here and put it away until someone can be called who is able to read a thermometer. At her first opportunity, she should learn how to read the thermometer herself.

When reading the thermometer:

1. Make sure the light is adequate for accurate reading of the thermometer.

2. Hold the thermometer by the top, in line with the eye; turn the ridged side toward you.

3. Look for the thin column of mercury between the lines and numbers through the ridge. It may be necessary to roll the thermometer slowly back and forth to locate the mercury; the end of the mercury column indicates the temperature.

4. Read the scale to include the degree and nearest two-tenths of a degree.

When shaking down the mercury:

1. Stand away from the furniture to avoid striking the thermometer against any object and breaking it.

2. Hold the thermometer firmly by the top between the thumb and first two fingers.

3. Shake with a loose wrist movement—as though shaking water off the hand—to bring the mercury to 95° F. or below.

Taking the Mouth Temperature

Equipment

Clinical thermometer

Container of wipes: absorbent cotton, paper tissues, toilet paper, or pieces of clean gauze or rags

Soap

Waste container

Container of cool, clean water

Procedure

1. Have the patient sit or lie down.

2. Hold the thermometer firmly by the top.

3. Shake the mercury down to 95° F. or below. (*See* explanation above.)

4. Rinse the thermometer in clear, cool water to make it easier and more pleasant to hold in the mouth.

5. Place the bulb in the patient's mouth, well under the tongue and a little to one side.

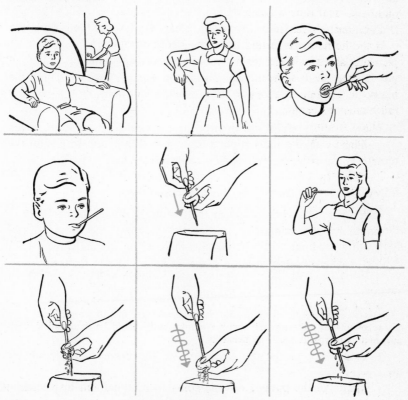

Taking temperature by mouth.

6. Instruct the patient to keep his lips closed, to breathe through his nose, and not to bite down on the thermometer or to talk.

7. Leave the thermometer in place for 3 minutes to assure an accurate registering.

8. Remove by holding at the top and use a wipe to remove any saliva; use a rotary motion from the top toward the bulb and over the bulb. This makes it easier to read. Dispose of the wipe in a waste container.

9. Take the thermometer to a good light, still holding by the top, and read.

10. Cleanse the thermometer immediately:

    a. Hold by the top, with the bulb down, over a waste container.

    b. Moisten a wipe with *cool* water and soap well. Beginning at the top, rub down with a single rotary stroke with friction, getting well into the grooves of the tube and over the bulb. Discard the wipe.

    c. Moisten a fresh wipe with clear, cool water and rinse the thermometer, using the same stroke as above.

    d. Soap and rinse again—repeat procedures *b* and *c*.

    e. Dry with a fresh wipe, using the same stroke, and put the thermometer away in its case, bulb end first.

11. Note the temperature on the daily record.

If there is any marked rise or drop in a patient's temperature, check the reading by taking the temperature again. Report the results to the doctor at once if the second reading confirms the first.

Taking the Rectal Temperature

The temperature of the body in the rectum is usually higher than in the mouth by approximately one degree; therefore, the normal rectal temperature is about 99.6° F. Always indicate on the daily record for the doctor when the temperature has been taken by the rectum.

Equipment

The same equipment will be needed as when taking a mouth temperature, with the exception that a thermometer with a stubby bulb should be used and a lubricant such as petrolatum will be needed.

Procedure for an Adult

1. Explain to the patient what is going to be done and instruct him to lie on his side.

2. Lubricate the bulb end of the thermometer with petrolatum, so that it will slide easily into the rectum. Any mild oil or cold cream may be used instead of petrolatum.

3. Slip the bulb end of the thermometer about 1 inch into the anus (opening of the rectum). *Hold in place* for 3 minutes to make sure the thermometer registers the actual temperature.

4. Remove the thermometer and follow directions *9* through *12* in Procedure for Taking the Mouth Temperature.

Procedure for an Infant or Child

1. Explain to the child what is going to be done, if he is old enough to understand.

2. Lubricate the thermometer in the same way as when taking the rectal temperature for an adult.

3. Have the child lie down (on his back or abdomen) on either the home nurse's lap, a bed, or a table.

4. Insert the bulb of the thermometer gently into the anus and hold it for 3 minutes. *It must be held in place at all times.* Help may be needed to hold a restless child.

5. Remove the thermometer and follow directions *9* through *12* in Procedure for Taking the Mouth Temperature.

Taking the Temperature by the Armpit

Temperature taken at the armpit is lower than the mouth temperature and should be recorded as taken in the armpit. To be reliable, it must be taken correctly. It may be ordered for infants and when other methods are difficult to follow. The same equipment will be needed as when taking a mouth temperature. Proceed as directed earlier in preparing the thermometer, except that the thermometer is not moistened.

Procedure

1. Dry the area under the arm.

2. Place the bulb of the thermometer in the armpit and have the patient press his arm firmly against his body with his hand on his opposite shoulder to hold the instrument in place. Leave the thermometer in this position for 10 minutes.

3. Remove the thermometer and read.

4. Cleanse the thermometer according to the directions in Procedure for Taking the Mouth Temperature.

5. Note the temperature and the manner of taking it on the daily record.

Essential Points To Remember.

1. Be sure the mercury is down to 95° F. or below before taking the temperature.

2. Allow sufficient time for an accurate registration of the temperature.

3. Take the temperature by the rectum or armpit when it cannot be taken accurately or safely by the mouth.

4. Cleanse the thermometer immediately after use.

TAKING THE PULSE AND RESPIRATION

Purpose. To count the pulse (number of heart beats) and respirations (breathing) that occur each minute.

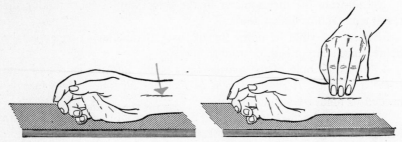

Locating wrist pulse.

Procedure

Pulse. 1. Have the patient lie or sit down. Place his arm and hand in a relaxed position, thumb up, supported on a chair arm, table, or bed.

2. Locate the pulse by placing the forefinger on the thumb side of the patient's wrist between the tendons and the wrist bone.

3. Count the pulse beats for 1 full minute; then check the rate by counting for another minute.

4. Note on the daily record for the doctor the pulse rate per minute, time, date, and any irregularity noted.

Respiration. Respirations may be counted immediately following the counting of the pulse and while the fingers are still on the pulse, as the patient is then less likely to be aware that the count is being made and to change his breathing.

1. Observe the rise and fall of the chest. Count for 1 full minute each rise of the chest.

2. Note on the daily record the rate and any unusual condition in breathing.

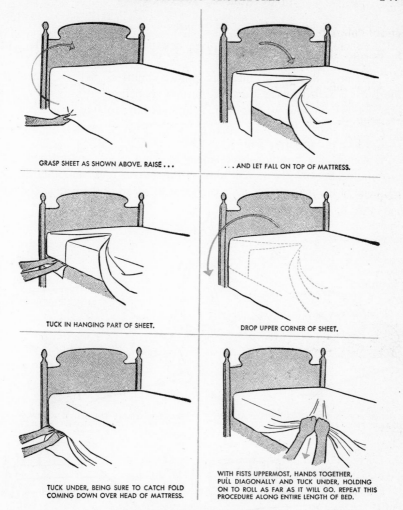

GRASP SHEET AS SHOWN ABOVE. RAISE . . .

. . . AND LET FALL ON TOP OF MATTRESS.

TUCK IN HANGING PART OF SHEET.

DROP UPPER CORNER OF SHEET.

TUCK UNDER, BEING SURE TO CATCH FOLD COMING DOWN OVER HEAD OF MATTRESS.

WITH FISTS UPPERMOST, HANDS TOGETHER, PULL DIAGONALLY AND TUCK UNDER, HOLDING ON TO ROLL AS FAR AS IT WILL GO. REPEAT THIS PROCEDURE ALONG ENTIRE LENGTH OF BED.

CHANGING THE BED LINEN

Purpose. To make a bed which provides for the patient safety, comfort, warmth, a smooth, clean surface to lie on, and freedom of movement.

Without the Patient in Bed

Equipment

Bed—comfortable and single, if possible
Firm, smooth mattress and pad
Clean sheets and pillow cases
Blankets, suited to room temperature
Pillows

Spread, lightweight
Extra sheet for a draw sheet with a waterproof sheet or pad to protect the mattress if necessary
Newspapers or a laundry bag for soiled linen

Procedure

1. Assemble the fresh linen; place newspapers or a bag to receive the soiled linen.

2. Remove the spread, blankets, pillows, mattress pad, and linen. If the linen is soiled, place it at once on newspapers or in a laundry bag; hold the bedding away from the face and clothing to avoid contact.

3. Turn the mattress.

4. Place the mattress pad.

5. Center the bottom sheet lengthwise and place on the bed. To anchor the bottom sheet well, allow 18 inches to tuck smoothly under the head of the mattress. Make a corner at the head of the bed, as shown.

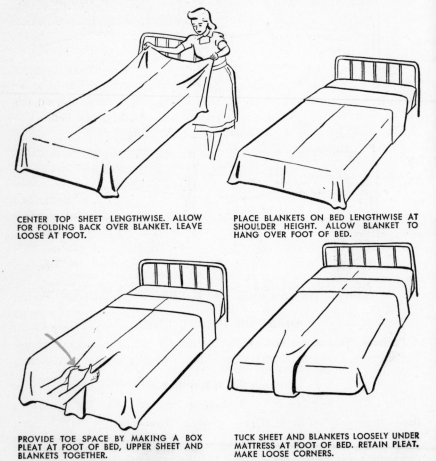

CENTER TOP SHEET LENGTHWISE. ALLOW FOR FOLDING BACK OVER BLANKET. LEAVE LOOSE AT FOOT.

PLACE BLANKETS ON BED LENGTHWISE AT SHOULDER HEIGHT. ALLOW BLANKET TO HANG OVER FOOT OF BED.

PROVIDE TOE SPACE BY MAKING A BOX PLEAT AT FOOT OF BED, UPPER SHEET AND BLANKETS TOGETHER.

TUCK SHEET AND BLANKETS LOOSELY UNDER MATTRESS AT FOOT OF BED. RETAIN PLEAT. MAKE LOOSE CORNERS.

Pleats provide space for toes.

6. Tuck the sheet smoothly under the mattress all the way down the side of the bed. If a draw sheet is used, fold it end to end and place *across* the center of the bed, with the top fold high enough to come under the pillow and the open end toward the foot; tuck under well. If additional protection is needed for the mattress, place a rubber sheet or substitute under the draw sheet.

7. Center the top sheet lengthwise and place. Allow enough to fold back over the blanket at the head of the bed and to tuck under the mattress at the foot of the bed. Leave loose at the foot until the blanket is in place.

8. Center the blanket lengthwise and place it at shoulder height. Leave loose at the foot of the bed. If the blanket is not long enough, two may be used, placing one blanket as desired to cover the shoulders and the other to tuck well under the mattress at the foot.

9. Go to the other side of the bed.

10. Tuck the lower sheet smoothly under the head of the mattress. Anchor it well by making a corner. Grip the sheet near the head of the bed; pull diagonally and tuck securely under the mattress. Repeat this three or four times all the way down the second side of the bed.

11. Pull the draw sheet smooth and tuck under.

12. Provide toe space.

13. Tuck the sheet and blankets loosely under the mattress at the foot of the bed; retain the pleat; make loose corners.

14. Center and place the bedspread. If the patient is using the bed at once, fold the spread under the upper edge of the blanket and fold the top sheet back over both the blanket and spread; tuck the bedspread loosely under the mattress at the foot.

15. Put on the pillow case. Keep the pillow away from the face and clothes.

16. Arrange the bed for occupancy. Fold the top covers—sheet, blankets, spread—in thirds to the foot of the bed with the free edge toward the head of the bed so the covers may be pulled up easily.

17. Remove the soiled linen.

With the Patient in Bed

Procedure

1. Assemble the equipment.

2. Loosen the bedding all around from under the mattress. Use care to avoid tearing.

3. Remove the spread; fold and hang over a chair. Remove one blanket, if using two; fold and hang over a chair. For the comfort of the patient, work from the head to the foot of the bed.

4. Remove the top sheet, sliding it down under the blanket. The patient may be asked to hold the top edge of the blanket while this is done, or the blanket can be tucked under the shoulders. If the top sheet is to be used as the bottom sheet or draw sheet, fold and place on a chair.

5. Remove all but one pillow—or all pillows. Remove the soiled cases and place with the soiled linen.

6. Turn the patient toward the other side of the bed in order to change the bottom sheet; keep him covered. (For procedures on turning the patient in bed, *see* p. 152.)

7. Change the bottom sheet.
   a. Gather the soiled bottom sheet lengthwise and roll it up close to the patient.
   b. Pull the mattress pad smooth under the patient.
   c. Center the clean sheet lengthwise; place and unfold, keeping about 18 inches to tuck under at the head to protect the mattress and to anchor the sheet.
   d. Gather the top half of the clean sheet and push in a flat roll *under* the soiled sheet, close up against the patient's back.
   e. Tuck the clean sheet well under the mattress at the head and make a corner; tuck well under the mattress all along the side of the bed. If a draw sheet is used, place on the bed with the folded edge under the pillow; tuck under the mattress.
   f. Turn the patient back toward the home nurse. Tell the patient what is about to be done. Loosen the blanket. Lift his feet over the soiled and clean sheets. Place one hand on his upper shoulder, the other on the upper hip on top of the bedding, and, *on signal,* roll the patient all the way toward the home nurse. Continue giving support while the bunched sheets are pulled out. Roll the patient on his back. Adjust the position and covers.
   g. Go to the other side of the bed and remove the soiled sheet, handling as little as possible; place with the soiled linen.
   h. Smooth the mattress pad.
   i. Adjust the clean bottom sheet. Tuck the sheet well under the mattress at the head of the bed; make a corner.

j. Tuck the sheet securely under the mattress all the way down the side of the bed, pulling the sheet diagonally.

k. Grasp and pull the draw sheet and tuck under the mattress.

8. Put on the clean pillow case and replace the pillow.

9. Place the top covers.

10. Make the patient comfortable; straighten the room and remove the soiled linen.

Essential Points To Remember.

1. The bottom sheet should be smooth and tight.

2. The top covers should be lightweight and suited to the temperature of the room, should provide for shoulder warmth and permit toe space, and should be held securely together.

3. Handle the soiled linen with care to prevent the spread of infection.

MOVING THE PATIENT IN BED

Purpose. To relax the patient, improve the circulation, prevent continued pressure on any part of the body over too long a time, avoid strain on the joints, prevent deformities, and adjust the position for comfort or for the giving of treatments.

Procedures

Helping the Patient Move to the Near Side of the Bed.

1. Place the hands, palms up, under the pillow, supporting the head and shoulders, and on signal pull toward the home nurse.

2. Place the hands, palms up, all the way under the hips and on signal pull toward the home nurse.

3. Place the hands under the knees and ankles, pull toward the home nurse, and adjust the body for position and comfort.

Helping the Patient Sit Up and Lie Down.

1. Face the head of the bed.

2. Flex the patient's knees.

3. Lock the near arms—the arm of the home nurse under the patient's arm with the hand braced at his shoulder; the patient's arm under her arm with his hand braced at her shoulder.

4. On signal, help the patient to a sitting position and pause in case he feels weak or dizzy.

5. Help the patient support himself, if he is able—hands braced back of him on the bed.

6. Lock arms as before and lower the patient to the pillow.

7. Adjust for correct position and comfort.

Helping the Patient Move Up and Down in Bed.

WHEN THE PATIENT CAN ASSIST.

1. Raise the patient to a sitting position as above.

2. Help the patient support himself—hands braced back of him on the bed.

3. Move toward the head of the bed—face the bed; place one hand low on the patient's back, the other, palm up, well under his thighs and on signal help the patient swing backward as he digs in and pushes with his heels.

4. Move toward the foot of the bed—repeat the same procedure except the patient digs in and pushes with his hands as he swings forward.

WHEN THE PATIENT IS HELPLESS.

If the patient is entirely helpless, two or even three people may be needed to lift him up or down in bed. For a single bed, two stand opposite each other and join hands under the patient's shoulders and thighs and move him as desired; for a double bed, two or three persons may work on the same side of the bed; one lifting the head and shoulders, one the hips, and one the legs and feet, supporting the knees and ankles. The drawsheet may also be used to help move or roll the patient.

Turning the Patient on His Side and Away from the Home Nurse.

1. Free the covers; instruct or help the patient to bend his knees.

2. Face the side of the bed, with one foot forward and the knees bent.

3. Slip one hand, palm up, all the way under the patient's shoulders; slip the other hand, palm up, all the way under the patient's hips. The home nurse bends at the hips and knees.

4. *On signal,* pull the patient toward the home nurse and roll him so that he is on his side.

5. Adjust the patient's hips, knees, and ankles for security and comfort.

6. Adjust the covers.

Turning the Patient Back from Side and Toward the Home Nurse.

1. Tell the patient what is about to be done.

2. Loosen the blanket.

3. Place one hand on the upper shoulder, the other on the upper hip on top of the bedding.

4. *On signal,* roll the patient all the way toward the home nurse.

5. Adjust the hips, knees, and ankles for comfort.

Essential Points To Remember.

1. Observe good posture.

2. Guide the patient's movements rather than do all the lifting.

PROVIDING SUPPORT FOR THE BED PATIENT

Purpose. To maintain correct and comfortable posture for the bed patient at all times.

Support for a Patient Lying on His Back

Equipment

Firm mattress and springs

Pillows—a variety, such as hard, soft, large, and small, or substitutes, as needed for the individual patient

Foot support—high enough to extend above the toes—to protect against the weight of the bedding

Procedure

The number and type of pillows under the head and shoulders is a matter of preference unless the doctor gives special orders. The normal curves of the spine should be maintained, the head in line with the trunk, i.e., not pushed forward or allowed to drop backward. The knees may be slightly bent for muscle relaxation and comfort.

Using One Pillow.

1. Place the pillow under the patient's head—reaching to the shoulders.

2. Place a foot support for his upright feet to brace against; it should extend above the toes to protect them from the weight of the bedding. (*See* Providing a Footrest, p. 208.)

3. Place a small pillow or folded towel under the knees as desired.

Using Three Pillows.

1. Place two lengthwise, overlapping at the top, together at the bottom, and extending under the shoulders.

2. Place one crosswise at the top under the head. (Place a small support at the lower back, if necessary.)

3. Place the foot and knee supports as above.

Support for a Patient Lying on His Side

Procedure

1. Place one pillow under the patient's head.
2. Place one snugly and securely at his back.
3. Place one lengthwise between his legs and feet, supporting the knee, toes, and heel; adjust the position of his legs for comfort by flexing the uppermost leg beyond the knee of the lower leg.
4. Place a small support under his abdomen.
5. Place one pillow for support of the uppermost arm. (The arm should be in line with the trunk, and the elbow in line with the shoulder.)

Support for a Patient Sitting Up in Bed

The doctor will indicate when the patient may sit up in bed and for how long.

Equipment

Back rest	Small pillow
Large pillows, 2–5	Foot support

Procedure

1. Place the back rest, slanting the surface toward the patient.
2. Adjust 3 pillows as described previously.
3. Swing the patient back to the pillows and help him lie back. (*See* Procedure for Moving the Patient in Bed.)
4. Place the knee support (a small pillow).
5. Place the foot support.
6. Place a pillow at either side for an arm support.
7. Note on the daily record the length of time the patient sat up and his reaction.

Essential Points To Remember.

1. Change the position from time to time.
2. Maintain correct body alignment.
3. Provide support to avoid strain on the joints, prevent deformities, conserve energy, and promote comfort.

HELPING THE PATIENT FROM THE BED TO A CHAIR AND BACK INTO BED

Purpose. To help stimulate circulation, provide relief from lying in bed, and promote general convalescence.

The doctor will indicate when the patient may sit up in a chair and for how long.

Equipment

Comfortable chair

Blankets, pillows, and footstool, as needed

Dressing gown, hose, and slippers

Extra shawl or wrap, if desired

Blocks for a wheelchair, if required

Preparation

1. Bring the chair near the bed, braced against a wall or other means of support. If a rocking chair or wheelchair is used, blocks will be needed to steady the chair unless an assistant is present.

2. Place the blankets and pillows as needed.

3. Have a footstool handy.

Procedure

Getting the Patient Out of Bed.

1. Help the patient to a sitting position; pause in case he shows signs of dizziness; have him support himself with his hands braced behind. With one hand on the small of the patient's back and the other under his knees, swing the patient, on signal, to allow his legs to hang over the edge of the bed. After abdominal surgery, to prevent strain, first roll the patient toward the home nurse on his side; place one hand under his head and lower shoulder, and one hand back of his knees; the patient places his uppermost hand on the home nurse's shoulder. Raise the patient and swing his legs over the edge of the bed.

2. Put the dressing gown, hose, and slippers on the patient.

3. Face the patient; place one foot forward, legs apart for balance; bend at the hips and knees.

4. Place the patient's hands on the home nurse's hips and grasp the patient's arms at the shoulders from the outer surface.

5. On signal, help the patient slide off the bed to stand on his feet; pause in case he feels dizzy.

6. Still supporting the patient, side-step to the chair, turning the patient so that he can feel the chair at the back of his legs.

7. On signal, help the patient sit down. Stand close to the patient, feet apart, one foot forward; bend the hips and knees to prevent back strain and help him lower himself into the chair.

8. Arrange the pillows, blankets, and footstool for comfort.

While the patient is in the chair, the bed may be aired, the mattress turned, and the bed remade with fresh linen.

Getting the Patient Back to Bed.

1. Open the bed—fan fold the upper bedding in thirds to the foot of the bed with the free end toward the head of the bed.

2. Release the blanket about the patient.

3. Face the patient, standing close to him with one foot forward, legs apart and braced for balance. Have the patient put the same foot forward and place his hands on the home nurse's hips. Grasp the patient's arms at the shoulders; bend the hips and knees, and, on signal, help the patient to a standing position. Pause in case he becomes dizzy.

4. Still supporting the patient, side-step to the bed.

5. Lift the dressing gown and help the patient to a sitting position on the edge of the bed with his hands braced behind for support.

6. Remove the dressing gown, hose, and slippers.

7. On signal, swing the patient back into bed, keeping one hand on the small of his back and one under his knees. Help him lie down.

8. Cover the patient and allow him to rest.

9. Note on the daily record the length of time the patient was up in the chair and his reactions to the experience.

Essential Points To Remember.

1. Before getting the patient up, obtain assistance if needed.

2. Place the chair near the bed the first day so the patient can be returned to bed quickly if necessary.

3. Protect the chair against slipping.

4. Avoid chilling and fatigue.

GIVING A BED BATH

Purpose. To cleanse, refresh, and relax the patient; stimulate circulation; provide a mild form of exercise; and aid in elimination by cleansing the pores.

Mouth care or treatments may be given before the bath.

Equipment

Large basin of *warm* water
Container of *hot* water
Waste water pail if not near a bathroom
Waste paper container
Towels—2 bath, 1 face
Washcloth
Soap in a dish
Lightweight or bath blanket
Rubbing alcohol (warmed)

Oil (sweet or mineral)
Body powder
Hand lotion and deodorant, if needed
Tray with toilet articles such as a hairbrush, comb, nail file, toothbrush, and mouthwash or dentifrice
Newspapers for protection of the furniture
Clean pajamas or gown
Clean bed linen

Preparation

1. See that the room is warm and that privacy is assured.

2. Assemble the equipment.

3. Remove and fold the spread.

4. Remove the top sheet—if soiled put on a newspaper or in a laundry bag; if to be used again, fold and place on the back of a chair.

5. Replace the regular blanket with a bath blanket if desired. Keep the patient well covered with a hot water bag to the feet if cold.

6. Remove all but one pillow unless ordered by the doctor.

7. Remove the soiled pillow cases; place with other soiled linen.

8. Remove the patient's gown or pajamas.

Procedure

1. Face.

    a. Place a towel under the head to protect the bedding. Place another towel across the patient's chest and tuck half-way under the top edge of the blanket.

    b. Wet the washcloth. Make a bath mitt by wrapping the cloth around the palm of the hand, anchoring with the thumb and tucking in the ends. Squeeze the cloth to prevent dripping.

    c. Wash the eyes gently from the nose toward the ear, using one corner of the mitt for one eye and the other corner for the other eye. Use no soap.

    d. Wash the forehead, nose, and cheeks, using firm, even pressure, long strokes, and an S-motion around the mouth and chin. Use soap if desired.

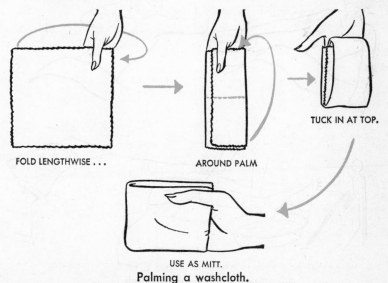

FOLD LENGTHWISE . . .   AROUND PALM   TUCK IN AT TOP.

USE AS MITT.

Palming a washcloth.

e. Rinse the face, following the same stroke as for washing.

f. Dry the face, following the same order and using the same stroke as in washing and rinsing. Wrap a section of the towel around the hand for a firm stroke and to avoid dragging the ends.

2. Ears and front of the neck.

a. Wash with soap and water, handling the washcloth in the same way as for washing the face. Get well into the folds of skin.

b. Rinse and dry.

3. Chest.

a. Cover the chest with a towel. Turn back the blanket protected with the towel.

b. Soap, rinse, and dry. Observe the skin; if it is reddened under the breasts, use a little body powder or oil.

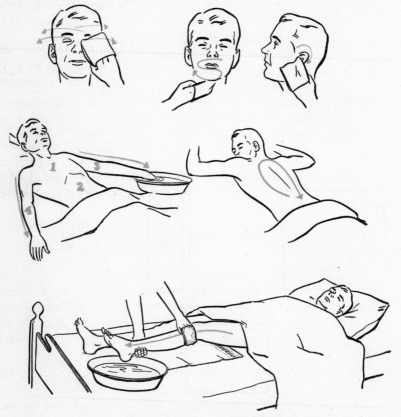

Steps in giving a bed bath.

4. Abdomen.
   a. Protect the blanket with a towel; leave one towel over the chest.
   b. Soap, rinse, and dry the abdomen, sides of trunk, and well over the upper thighs and pubic area. Use firm strokes.
   c. Pull up the blanket and remove the towels.

5. Arm.
   a. Place one towel under the arm and shoulder; place the other back over the blanket and tuck under the edge lengthwise.
   b. Soap, rinse, and dry the arm. Be sure to include the armpit area. Give support to the arm while washing it.

6. Hand.
   a. Place a basin of water and a dish of soap securely at the patient's side on a towel.
   b. Soap, wash, and rinse the patient's hand in the basin. Remove the basin and soap. Dry thoroughly.
   c. Clean the nails; apply hand lotion, if necessary.

7. Other arm and hand. Repeat the procedure in the same way with the other arm and hand. Work from the same side of the bed. Keep the water warm by adding hot water. Change the water whenever necessary (soiled or too soapy).

8. Back of neck, back, and buttocks.
   a. Roll the patient on his side away from the person giving the bath. (*See* p. 152.) Fold back the blanket to uncover his back.
   b. Protect the bedding; place one towel on the bottom sheet close to the back and one over the blanket, tucked under the free edge.
   c. Soap, rinse, and dry, using long, firm strokes. Examine for reddened areas due to pressure. Follow with a back rub. (*See* p. 160.) Relieve the pressure by the use of an air cushion or a "donut," if necessary. (*See* p. 212.)

9. Leg.
   a. Keep the patient covered except for the part being washed. Wrap the blanket snugly at the groin; protect the bedding with towels.
   b. Have the patient bend his knee. Support the leg; wash, rinse, and dry with long, firm strokes. Examine the skin, especially the knee, for reddened or roughened areas and apply oil if needed.

10. Foot.
   a. Protect the bed near the foot with newspapers and a towel. Place the basin and dish of soap securely on a towel.
   b. Lift the foot carefully into the basin; wash and rinse the foot with firm strokes.

    c. Remove the foot from the basin and dry, especially between the toes. If the skin is dry, apply oil. If the heel is sore, relieve the pressure with a "donut."

    d. Remove the towels and cover the leg.

11. Other leg and foot. Repeat the same procedure with the other leg and foot, working from the same side of the bed.

12. Genitals.

    a. The patient may wash his genitals, if able. Place a dry towel under the buttocks to protect the bedding. Place the basin handy for the patient; give him the soaped washcloth and a bath towel.

    b. If the patient is unable to do this, cleanse the genitals. If genital discharges are present, use absorbent cotton or soft tissues and burn them later. Special care may be advised by the doctor following childbirth.

    c. Remove the towel; arrange the blanket.

13. Replace the gown or pajamas.

14. Comb the hair (*see* p. 172). If the patient is a woman, she may wish to put on make-up.

15. Straighten the bed.

16. Remove and clean all bath equipment.

17. Arrange the bedside table.

18. Note on the daily record any unusual conditions observed. These may include reddened areas due to pressure, rash, swelling, unusual lumps, sores, or a tendency to fatigue.

Essential Points To Remember.

1. Cleanse all parts of the body.

2. Avoid chilling, fatigue, or embarrassment of the patient.

3. Observe and report to the doctor any unusual conditions.

THE BACK RUB

Purpose. To refresh and relax the patient, stimulate blood circulation, and relieve pressure.

Equipment

Rubbing alcohol, warmed in a container of hot water, or oil   Body powder, if desired

Procedure

1. Warm the hands; trim the nails short enough to avoid scratching the patient.

2. Place the patient comfortably on his side, facing away from the nurse, or on his stomach.

3. Pour a small amount of warmed rubbing alcohol or oil on the hands for lubrication.

4. Stand facing the head of the bed with one foot slightly forward and the knees slightly bent. Then with the flat of both hands and with long, firm, continuous strokes, apply pressure up and down the entire back, including the shoulders, back, and buttocks. Keep the hands lubricated so they will glide comfortably over the body. As the hands move up and down the back, the home nurse swings forward and backward with her knees bent.

5. Observe the condition of the skin and give additional massage where there are reddened areas. Such areas may indicate impaired circulation due to pressure. Pay special attention to the base of the spine and to the shoulder blades.

6. A small amount of talcum on the hands can be used to finish the rub. (Avoid powder crumbs in the bed.)

7. Assist the patient to a comfortable position after the back rub.

8. Report to the doctor any sign of broken skin or an unusually reddened area.

Essential Points To Remember.

1. Have the patient in a comfortable position and avoid chilling.

2. Use a stroke firm enough to relax the muscles yet gentle enough for soothing comfort, continue long enough to be effective.

3. Report to the doctor any unusual condition of the skin.

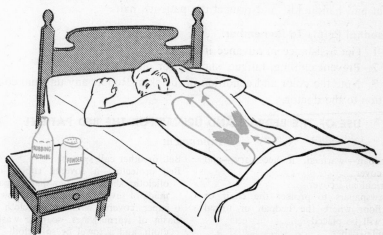

Use long firm strokes in giving a back rub.

TUB BATH FOR THE CONVALESCENT, HANDICAPPED, OR ELDERLY PATIENT

Purpose. To give a cleansing bath with safety, comfort, and minimum exertion for the patient who is able to use the bathroom facilities.

Equipment

Washcloth

Towels

Soap

Fresh clothing, warmed if necessary

Blanket, if needed

Chair or stool covered with a pad and placed beside the tub

Bathmat in front of a chair

Rubber suction mat for the tub

Bath seat, if desired

Bathtub one-quarter to one-half full of comfortably warm water

Glass of cool water in case the patient feels faint

Procedure

1. Collect the equipment and draw the water.

2. Assist the patient to the warmed bathroom; help him undress.

3. Help the patient into the tub. Have him grasp some secure object and give him support.

4. Soap and rinse well, rubbing the body briskly but gently all over to promote circulation.

5. Drain the tub and assist the patient to a chair. Protect him from chilling and help him dry his body thoroughly.

6. Assist the patient to dress and return to his room. Suggest that he rest quietly.

7. Clean the tub and straighten the bathroom.

If a shower bath is preferred, care should be taken to adjust the temperature of the water before the patient enters the bath, provide a floor mat and handholds, and protect the patient's hair.

Essential Points To Remember.

1. Get assistance in advance if needed.

2. Prevent chilling, fatigue, slipping, or other accidents.

3. Note the color and condition of the skin. Report any unusual condition to the doctor.

USE OF THE BEDPAN AND URINAL FOR THE BED PATIENT

Equipment

Bedpan—warmed, if necessary—and cover

Urinal and cover

Newspapers to protect the chair or floor where the bedpan or urinal will be placed

Toilet paper

Bell or other call system

Bed protector—a covered rubber or oilcloth sheet or newspaper pad made of several thicknesses of newspapers covered with a clean cloth

Basin of warm water, soap, a washcloth, and a towel or soft cloth

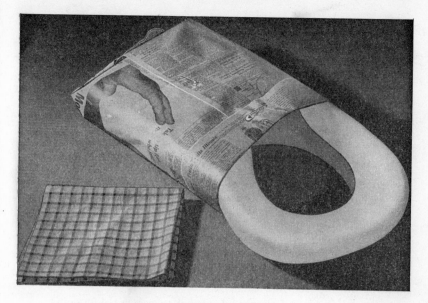

Bedpan and covers.

Procedure

Giving the Bedpan.

1. Bring the covered bedpan, the pad for bed protection, the toilet paper, and the bell to the room.

2. Place the pad under the patient's hips.

3. Fold back the covers at the side to prevent soiling.

4. Place the bedpan on the bed beside the patient; grasp by the side or closed end and have the open end toward the foot of the bed.

5. Place one hand under the small of the patient's back and on signal help the patient lift his hips; with the other hand, slip the pan under the patient's hips and adjust for comfort. The patient may wish to be helped to a sitting position, if the doctor permits. Unless there is need to remain with the patient, place the toilet paper and call bell handy and leave the room.

6. Cleanse the patient after use of the pan; the patient does this if he is able. To avoid spreading the soiled area to the openings of bladder and vagina, wipe downward toward the spine.

7. Remove the pan in the same manner as placed.

8. Observe the skin for redness or soreness. Keep the skin dry.

9. Observe the contents of the pan and note on the daily record. If unusual, save for the doctor to see.

10. Clean the pan.
   a. Empty it into the toilet, unless the doctor has ordered otherwise.
   b. Rinse with cold water (this helps prevent the stool from sticking to the pan).
   c. If necessary, loosen the particles of stool with a toilet paper wad; wash thoroughly with hot soapy water and rinse.
   d. Wipe dry and put away.
11. Provide for the patient to cleanse his hands.

Giving the Urinal.

Help the patient place the urinal, if necessary. Remove promptly after use. Note the content and cleanse thoroughly. Keep covered before and after use.

Using a Commode.

(*see* Making Substitute Equipment, p. 202)

1. Help the patient out of bed to the commode (*see* Helping the Patient from the Bed to a Chair).
2. Provide robe and slippers if needed to prevent chilling.
3. Give assistance back to bed.
4. Note the content, and cleanse as for the bedpan.
5. It is very important that the commode, which may be kept at the bedside, be clean and free from odors.

Essential Points To Remember.

1. Avoid injury to the patient by lifting his hips high enough to prevent his skin from rubbing against the pan.
2. Offer the bedpan or urinal at intervals even though the patient does not request it and give promptly whenever desired.

MEASURING URINE OUTPUT
Measuring Twenty-four-hour Output

Purpose. To determine the total amount of urine being passed throughout the entire twenty-four-hour period.

The amount of urine passed depends largely on the amount of liquid taken into the body, and the doctor usually wishes liquid intake measured and recorded also.

Equipment

Measuring container, marked in ounces   Bedpan or urinal
if possible, kept for this purpose
alone—commercial or homemade—
a tin can, jar, or other container

Procedure

1. Instruct the patient that the urine is being measured and that the bedpan should not be used at the same time for both bowel movement and urine.

2. Empty the contents of the pan or urinal into the measuring container and record the amount in ounces after each time urine is passed.

3. Cleanse the equipment.

If the patient is using a urinal, the measurements may already be marked on it, or the home nurse may mark the urinal with strips of adhesive tape measuring the amounts exactly in ounces. If the patient is able to go to the toilet, place a bedpan or basin on the toilet seat, and after use measure the contents.

Collecting a Specimen (Sample) of Urine

Purpose. To provide a single specimen of urine for examination.

When a specimen of urine is requested by the doctor, ask him how much he needs and when he wishes it taken. It is usual to take a specimen from the first urine passed in the morning unless a twenty-four-hour specimen is requested, and 4 to 6 ounces is usually sufficient. The patient should understand that the specimen of urine should be kept separate from a bowel movement.

Equipment

Clean bedpan, urinal, or other receptacle

Clean bottle large enough for the specimen ordered by the doctor—with a watertight stopper

Label to be attached to the bottle, giving the following information: "Urine"—name of the patient, date, and hour

Procedure

1. Wash the patient's genitals before urine is passed or have the patient do this if he goes to the bathroom. (If the patient is menstruating or has a discharge, report this to the doctor before the specimen is collected.)

2. The patient urinates into a clean receptacle.

3. Transfer the urine to the specimen bottle and cork securely. Fill in the label and attach to the bottle.

4. Make the specimen available to the doctor as promptly as possible.

5. Cleanse the equipment as usual.

Collecting a Twenty-four-hour Specimen of Urine

Purpose. To provide a specimen from the total twenty-four-hour output of urine.

If the doctor wants all urine passed by the patient to be *saved* (so that he may get a twenty-four-hour specimen), the patient must wash the genitals each time before passing urine. Begin at a stated hour—usually 7 A.M.; discard the first urine passed at this hour. Pour all urine passed thereafter into a large clean vessel—a large chamber or enamel pail will do. Save all the urine passed up to *and* including that passed at 7 A.M. the next morning. Keep the vessel tightly covered. The urine may then be measured (if ordered) and a sample collected from this total amount, usually 4 to 6 ounces.

Essential Points To Remember.

1. Cleanliness of the receptacles and genitals.
2. Accuracy in measurement and labeling.

GIVING AN ENEMA

Purpose. To aid in elimination and to rid the lower bowel of waste material.

To an Adult

Equipment

Tray for the equipment

Enema bag, can, or fountain syringe (If a fountain syringe is not available, the solution may be made in a pitcher and poured into a funnel to which the soft rectal tube or catheter used as a nozzle is attached)

Connecting tubing, stopcock, and enema nozzle

Enema solution, as ordered by the doctor (If he does not specify, give 1 pint of plain warm water)

Lubricant for the nozzle

Toilet paper

Warmed bedpan and cover, unless the patient uses the toilet

Bed protection—a rubber sheet, oilcloth, or bed pad

Extra blanket

Basin of warm water, washcloth, and towel

Newspapers for protection of the furniture

Call bell

Standard on which to hang the enema bag—a floor lamp, stepladder, or hatrack

All equipment should be clean and tested for leaks, and the stopcock should be checked to be sure it is in working order.

The room should be warm and free from drafts; the door should be closed for privacy.

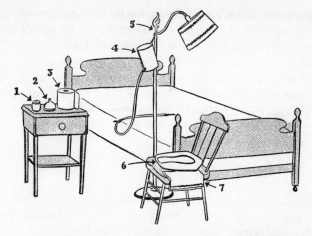

1. PETROLATUM. 2. CALL BELL. 3. TOILET PAPER. 4. CONTAINER, TUBING, STOPCOCK, AND ENEMA TIP. OUTFLOW OF CONTAINER SHOULD BE 12" TO 18" ABOVE MATTRESS. 5. FLOOR LAMP OR SUITABLE STANDARD. 6. BEDPAN ON PROTECTED AREA. 7. BEDPAN COVER.

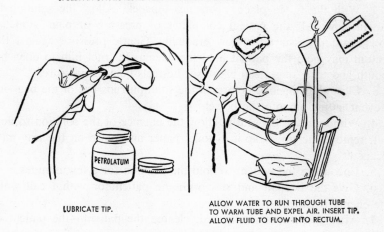

LUBRICATE TIP.

ALLOW WATER TO RUN THROUGH TUBE TO WARM TUBE AND EXPEL AIR. INSERT TIP. ALLOW FLUID TO FLOW INTO RECTUM.

Preparing to give an enema.

Preparation

1. Protect the table and chair. Have a bedpan handy.

2. Cover the patient with the extra blanket. Fold back the upper bedclothes and place over the chair at the foot of the bed.

3. Have the patient at the near side of the bed and place the bed protection under his hips.

4. Roll up the gown or remove the pajama trousers.

5. The patient may lie on his side or on his back; one pillow or none.

6. Hang the bag so that the outlet is about 12 to 18 inches above the upper surface of the mattress, assuring a gentle flow.

7. Close the stopcock and pour the solution into the bag.

8. Open the stopcock and allow a little solution to flow into the bedpan to make sure the air is out of the tubing. Test the temperature of the solution on the wrist; it should be comfortably warm. Close the stopcock.

9. Lubricate the nozzle.

Procedure

1. Insert the enema tip into the anus about 2 to 3 inches and hold in place. The patient may wish to do this. If there is blocking, rotate the tip slightly, but gently; withdraw it a little and try again. It may become clogged. If clogged, withdraw the tip; allow the solution to run through; insert again.

2. With the tip in place, open the stopcock. Allow the solution to run in slowly. If the patient complains of pressure or pain, stop the flow; wait; then start the flow gradually. Gentle pressure against the rectum may help the patient hold the enema. Instruct him to open his mouth and take long, deep breaths if he feels pain or pressure.

3. Close the stopcock before all the solution runs out of the bag—to prevent letting air into the bowel.

4. Withdraw the tip gently; allow the balance of the solution to flow out; remove the tip; wrap it in toilet paper and place on the tray until cleaned.

5. Encourage the patient to hold the solution for a few minutes.

6. Give the bedpan and stay with the patient or within call while the enema is expelled.

7. After the enema is expelled, cleanse the patient—the patient or nurse may do this. Dry thoroughly.

8. Remove the bedpan and cover immediately.

9. Remove the bed protection; replace the upper bedclothes; make the patient comfortable. Air the room but do not chill the patient.

10. See that the patient's hands are washed if he has helped with giving the enema.

11. Note the contents of the bedpan; if unusual, save for the doctor to see. Note also the patient's reaction.

12. Care for the equipment.

    a. Empty the bedpan; cleanse and put away.

b. Open the stopcock; rinse the bag and tubing with clear water; hang to drain. When dry, replace in its box or wrap in a clean cloth; leave the stopcock open. If an enema bag is used, stuff it with tissue paper to keep the sides from sticking together. Keep dry.

c. Scrub the enema nozzle with hot soapy water; rinse; boil 3 minutes; dry and place with the bag.

To a Child

The room should be warm and free from drafts.

A child may lie on a well-protected bed on his back or side.

If the enema is given on the home nurse's lap, the rubber sheet and diaper should cover her clothes. A folded towel placed under the buttocks will raise them slightly to the right level to receive the enema.

If the child is old enough, explain what is going to be done and proceed to give the enema as described for an adult, giving the solution very slowly and with a gentle flow. Give the amount ordered by the doctor, usually about one-half pint.

Cleansing or Oil Enema for a Baby

Equipment

Small rubber bulb syringe with a nozzle

Warm water or oil for the enema (the doctor will order the amount)

Toilet paper

Small basin or chamber to receive the enema

Small blanket for warmth

Rubber sheet, oilcloth, or newspapers covered with a diaper to protect the home nurse's lap

Basin of warm water and a soft washcloth for cleansing

Clean diapers

Procedure

1. Place the baby on his back on the lap or on a well-protected table. Remove his diapers. Fold back his clothes.

2. Take up the warm water or oil in the syringe, holding the nozzle up, and squeeze the bulb gently to expel air. Test the temperature of the liquid on the inner surface of the wrist. It should be comfortably warm.

3. Lift the baby's legs with one hand, holding at the ankles with a finger between them. Be sure the liquid is still in point of nozzle (to avoid injecting air). Gently insert the nozzle of the syringe about an inch into the anus.

4. Give the water or oil by very gently and slowly squeezing the bulb of the syringe. A small baby will usually take about 2 or 3 ounces, an older baby more.

5. When the syringe is empty, withdraw it carefully and place on toilet paper. Press the baby's buttocks together with a folded diaper to help the baby hold the enema for a few minutes.

6. Place the edge of the basin or chamber under the baby's hips to receive the bowel movement. If the enema is expelled without a bowel movement, a second may be given.

7. After the bowels have moved, wash the baby with warm water; dry him thoroughly; put on a fresh diaper and put him back to bed.

8. Care for the equipment after use.
  a. Note the appearance of the stool and inform the doctor of any unusual condition. Cleanse the chamber.
  b. Wash the syringe with hot soapy water; rinse with clear water and boil 5 minutes. Rinse, drain, and dry. Wrap in a clean cloth or paper and put away.

9. Note on the daily record the time the enema was given, the amount taken, the amount and character of the stool, such as undigested food, blood and mucus (jellylike liquid), and whether gas was expelled with the enema. Note the baby's condition after treatment.

Essential Points To Remember.

1. Assure a gentle flow of solution without pressure.

2. Select a good nozzle and lubricate well; avoid injury to the membrane.

3. Give no more solution than ordered by the doctor.

4. Have the patient lying down and in a comfortable position.

5. Avoid chilling.

GIVING CARE TO THE MOUTH

Purpose. To cleanse and refresh the patient's mouth, teeth, and gums; stimulate the circulation of the gums to keep them healthy; and prevent the accumulation of the brownish material (sordes) that sometimes collects in the mouths of sick people.

Bed Patient Who Is Able To Help Himself

Equipment

Small tray containing toothbrush, toothpaste or powder, or a glass of warm water to which has been added ½ teaspoonful each of salt and bicarbonate of soda or other mouthwash

Glass of clear, cool water
Small basin for the patient to spit into
Waste container
Towel or other protection

Procedure

1. Protect the bedding by placing a towel or other protection well up under the patient's chin, over the shoulders, and over the bedding.

2. If the patient is able to sit up, he may hold the basin in his lap and clean his teeth in the usual way, rinsing well with clear water.

3. If he is not able to sit up, turn his head to one side and place the basin near his chin. Pour water over the brush and apply dentifrice or the salt solution. Let the patient brush his teeth himself. Raise his head to help him take a mouthful of clear water, rinse, and spit out into the basin held for him under his chin. Repeat until the patient has finished.

Bed Patient Who Is Helpless
Equipment

Tray containing large-size cotton applicators
Lubricant for the lips
Glass of mouthwash or salt-soda solution

Glass of fresh water
Paper tissues
Towel or other protection
Small basin for the patient to spit into
Waste container

Procedure

1. Place a towel or other protection over the chest and shoulders, well up under the chin.

2. Examine the mouth, tongue, and gums carefully in a good light.

3. Moisten the applicator or swab, pressing out excess moisture against the side of the glass.

4. Steady the patient's chin with one hand and gently cleanse the mouth, gums, and teeth. Discard the applicator in a waste container. Cleanse one section of the mouth at a time and repeat with clean applicators until the entire mouth is clean. Cleanse the tongue.

5. Rinse, using fresh applicators dipped in clear water if the patient is unable to use the basin as in brushing the teeth.

6. Use an ointment or lubricant on the lips, if dry.

7. Remove the towels and tray. Dispose of waste material.

8. Note on the daily record any unusual condition found.

Essential Points To Remember.

1. Cleanse as often as needed for comfort and welfare.

2. Avoid injury to the membrane.

Care of Dentures (False Teeth)
Procedure

1. Ask the patient to remove his dentures and hand them to the nurse in a wipe.

2. Hold the teeth under running water, out of sight of the patient, handling with a wipe until one part is clean. Use a mild soap in cleansing them. If working over a wash basin, have the basin partly filled with cold water to lessen the danger of breakage should the denture slip out of the hand.

3. Rinse the teeth in cold water.

4. Rinse the patient's mouth with clear water or mouthwash.

5. Return the teeth lubricated with cool water to the patient, or place them in an opaque container in a safe place out of sight. Some types of dentures may be kept in water; others may not. Find out which type the patient has.

GIVING CARE TO THE PATIENT'S HAIR

Purpose. To cleanse and stimulate the hair and scalp and to make the patient more comfortable.

Daily care of the hair should be given to all patients. This may be done by brushing and combing. Occasionally a bed patient may need a shampoo. The services of a barber or a friend may be required at intervals to shave men patients unable to do this for themselves and to trim the hair for both men and women.

Equipment

Brush and comb   Hair tonic or cleanser,
Towel   if desired
Waste container

Procedure

Brushing and Combing the Hair of a Woman Patient.

1. Protect the bedding with a towel under the head.

2. Turn the head far to one side and part the hair all the way down the front and back.

3. Hold the strands of hair with the fingers between the scalp and the comb. Begin brushing at the ends and continue until the tangles are removed. Be sure to reach all portions of the scalp and hair. Lotions and creams are available that help loosen badly tangled hair.

4. Turn the head and repeat the same procedure.

5. Arrange the style as the patient wishes. If the patient is helpless, arrange in the most comfortable way to avoid tangles and inconvenience. For long hair, two braids are suggested.

6. Remove the towel and clean the equipment before putting it away.

7. Note on the daily record any unusual condition of the scalp or hair.

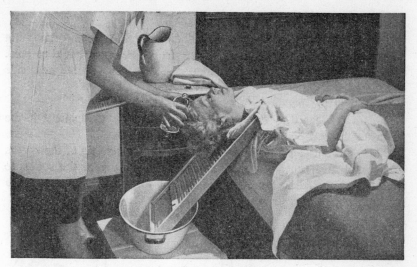

Shampoo time for the bed patient.

Washing the Hair of a Bed Patient.

The doctor may permit a patient to have a shampoo in bed. For this more or less infrequent service, a hairdresser may be called in for women patients. If such help is not available, the home nurse can give a satisfactory shampoo to a bed patient who is not critically ill. She should remember to wash the hair when the patient is rested and when a rest period can follow. The patient should be placed in a position that is comfortable and convenient, with the head slightly lowered. Place a towel around the patient's shoulders and provide protection for the bedding. Cleanse, rinse, and dry the hair thoroughly.

Essential Points To Remember.

1. Avoid fatigue and chilling.
2. Protect the surroundings.

FEEDING THE HELPLESS PATIENT

Purpose. To give nourishment to a helpless person in a way that will be enjoyable to him and encourage acceptance of food.

Equipment

Food as ordered, arranged attractively on a tray

Napkin or other protection
Drinking tube and silverware

Procedure

1. Test the food for temperature; liquids should be comfortably hot when tested on the home nurse's inner wrist. Cold foods should be cold.

2. See that the patient is in a comfortable position on the near side of the bed.

3. Protect the bedding; provide a napkin.

4. Bring a chair to the bedside and sit beside the patient if the height of the bed permits easy working; avoid hurry.

5. Give the first spoonful slowly; feed from the side tip of the spoon, a spoonful at a time; remove fluid from the bottom of the spoon to avoid dripping. Allow time for the patient to swallow. Do not leave spoon in liquid. It absorbs heat and may burn the patient.

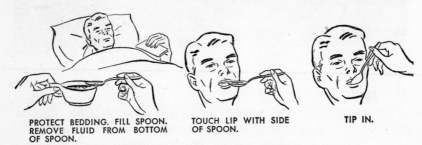

PROTECT BEDDING. FILL SPOON.   TOUCH LIP WITH SIDE   TIP IN.
REMOVE FLUID FROM BOTTOM   OF SPOON.
OF SPOON.

Feeding the helpless patient with a spoon.

6. When using a drinking tube, place it well into the liquid and hold for the patient. Stir the liquid; in the bottom of the cup it is likely to be hotter than on the surface.

7. When helping the patient drink from a cup, support his head with a hand under the pillow; hold the cup by the handle, but let the patient guide the cup and control the rate of flow by holding a hand on the bottom of the cup.

8. Care of equipment: Rinse the tube in cold water; wash the dishes, silver, tray, and tube in hot soapy water; scald and drain dry.

9. Note on the daily record what the patient ate, at what time, and how much. Comment on his appetite and his enjoyment of the food.

Procedure for Feeding a Paralyzed or Semiconscious Patient

It is very important to be assured before feeding a semiconscious or paralyzed patient that he is able to swallow; give very small amounts and be sure the patient has swallowed before feeding more. Only liquids are given and usually they are warm, never hot.

1. Test the liquid on the inner surface of the wrist.

2. Move the patient to the near side of the bed and raise his head on the pillow. Protect the bedding and gown.

3. Sit beside the bed, if the height of the bed permits ease in working.

4. Turn the patient's head slightly to one side and feed slowly, a half teaspoonful at first or a few drops with a medicine dropper. Put the liquids well back in the mouth.

5. Wait until the patient swallows before feeding more. Keep the lips and chin clean.

6. Rinse with water and wipe the mouth after feeding.

7. Adjust the patient to a comfortable position.

8. Note on the daily record the amount and kind of food taken by the patient and at what time.

Essential Points To Remember.

1. A calm, unhurried manner is important in getting the patient's coöperation.

2. Serve small amounts at a time and be sure the patient can swallow to avoid strangling.

3. Avoid burning—be sure the liquid is only comfortably hot.

WASHING DISHES AND EATING UTENSILS

Purpose. To cleanse dishes and so avoid transfer of disease.

When there is illness, the strictest cleanliness should be observed in the care of articles used by the patient; therefore, dishwashing deserves special attention. Soap, hot water, and friction properly applied will offer reasonable safeguards for the care of dishes and silver. In some circumstances, the doctor may order boiling.

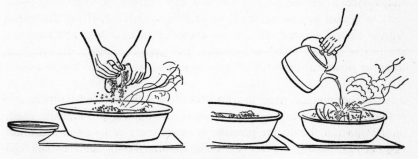

Effective dishwashing.

Equipment

Receptacles for washing and scalding
   the dishes
Rack for draining, or a clean towel
Clean dishcloth

Hot water
Soap or some other detergent (a water
   softener if needed)

Procedure

1. Scrape the dishes and stack.
2. Dispose of all food from the invalid's tray (put liquids into a waste pail or toilet; wrap solids securely and burn or place in the garbage).
3. Prepare hot soapy water in a dishpan (an amount sufficient to cover the dishes well).
4. Wash, rubbing well, especially where the patient's mouth has touched, such as the rims of cups and glasses, the bowls of spoons, and between the tines of forks.
5. Rinse well with scalding water.
6. Dry with a clean towel or place in a rack to drain.

GIVING MEDICINES

Purpose. To administer medication correctly to promote the recovery or welfare of the patient.

If the doctor writes a prescription (a written order over his signature), it is taken to a druggist to be filled. The druggist fills the prescription and usually includes the following information on the label of the container: name of the patient, name of the doctor, date filled, instructions for taking, and the prescription number.

Medicine by Mouth. Medicines may be in the form of liquids, powders, pills, tablets, or capsules. They may be ordered to be taken only once, once a day or several times a day, before or after meals—in fact, on almost any schedule. Take or give as ordered. If the directions are not clearly understood, call the doctor. Powders, pills, and capsules are nearly always given with water. Powders are either dissolved in water or placed at the back of the tongue and washed down with water. If the pill or capsule is placed well back on the tongue, a swallow of water taken, and the head thrown back, it will usually roll down easily.

Disagreeable medicine may be followed by a cookie, cracker, fruit, or fruit juice if the doctor permits, but care must be taken in this practice because patients—especially children—may associate the food with the medicine and so acquire a distaste for the food. A drinking tube or straw may be used in taking disagreeable medicine or when the medicine may discolor the teeth.

Medicine by Hypodermic Injection. The doctor occasionally wishes medicine given by hypodermic injection—the medicine in liquid form is injected under the skin through a needle—but unless he or a professional registered nurse teaches someone in the family or the patient himself to give the medicine in this way, it should never be attempted. The public health nurse or the visiting nurse will be glad to teach a member of the family if the doctor gives his permission.

Other Methods of Giving Medicine. There are other ways of giving medicine, such as by inhalation (*see* Inhalations and Throat Irrigations, p. 188), by rectum, by absorption through the skin, and directly into the blood stream through injection into a vein. The last named will always be given by a doctor or professional nurse.

Giving Liquid Medicine to an Adult by Mouth
Equipment

On a tray:
  Medicine as ordered
  Medicine glass
  Standard-size teaspoon or medicine
    dropper
  Glass of fresh water

Paper tissue or napkin
Something to take away the taste, if
  desired and allowed, such as a piece
  of ice, a cracker, or a slice of orange

Procedure

1. Compare the label on the medicine bottle with the doctor's orders —read aloud. Shake well if ordered.

2. Remove the cork, placing it top side down on the tray.

3. Read the label again.

4. Pour the medicine into a spoon or medicine glass, holding the bottle with the label toward the palm to prevent soiling the label with medicine (this lessens the danger of mistakes). Measure the amount accurately. Hold the medicine glass so that the line measuring the needed amount is at eye level. If drops are given, count out loud. Avoid letting the solution run into the bulb of the dropper. Add water if allowed.

5. Give to the patient; follow by water or other "chaser," if allowed. Be sure the patient swallows the medicine. Cough syrups are not diluted and can be taken directly from a spoon.

6. Note on the daily record the kind and amount of medicine given,

the time, and any effects noted later. Also note if the patient was asleep or refused or vomited the medicine.

7. Care of equipment after use:
   a. Cleanse the glasses and spoon.
   b. Set up the tray ready for the next use and put in a safe place.

If tablets or pills are ordered, compare the label on the box with the doctor's orders; place the tablet in a spoon; close the box and read the label again before putting the box down. Give the tablet to the patient from the spoon. The tablet may be chewed or swallowed whole, according to order. Capsules and pills are usually swallowed whole and therefore cool, fresh water should be served with the capsule.

Medicines for Children

All that has been said about medicines in the preceding paragraphs applies to medicines prescribed for children as well as for adults.

A child may resist taking his medicine. The use of force or bribes with candy, toys, or money is undesirable. Instead, the child should be helped to understand that the medicine is necessary to help him get well and that the doctor, his father, or some other trusted person will be proud of him if he takes it without fuss. Some children respond quickly if they are made to feel that the decision to take medicine rests in their hands. Taking the medicine from a glass with a straw or from a special toy cup may appeal to a child.

If the child is not old enough to swallow a pill, tablet, or capsule, crush the pill or tablet or empty the capsule into a spoon; let it dissolve by adding just enough water to make a swallow. Follow the dose with another swallow or teaspoon of clear water.

Giving Medicine to a Baby

The equipment and procedure in giving medicine to a baby is much the same as for giving an adult liquid medicine except that it is usually given with a teaspoon or medicine dropper after it is diluted with water. A towel may be needed to protect the gown or bedding.

Essential Points To Remember.

1. A special prescription was meant for one person alone for conditions existing at the time it was prescribed. Do not give it to anyone else. Avoid self-dosage.
2. Give only when and as directed by the doctor.
3. Note and record any reaction to the medication.
4. Keep all medicines clearly labeled in a safe place away from chil-

dren and apart from other household bottles and jars; any drug may be unsafe if the wrong dosage is taken.

5. When giving medicine, have a good light; read the label aloud at least twice, once when taking the bottle from the shelf and once after the medicine is poured or the pill or capsule removed from the container.

6. If the medicine looks, smells, or tastes different from usual or if the pills are discolored or the liquid has crystallized, do not give it until the safety of use has been checked with the doctor.

7. Keep medicines that are put in dark bottles in a dark place—light affects them. Avoid freezing liquid medicines.

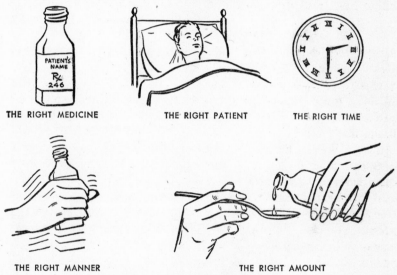

THE RIGHT MEDICINE   THE RIGHT PATIENT   THE RIGHT TIME

THE RIGHT MANNER   THE RIGHT AMOUNT

Five "rights" in giving medicine.

8. The adults in a family should all know where the medicines are kept. For emergency use, it is a good plan to have in a handy place the doctor's name and telephone number and the telephone number of the nearest hospital. A list of antidotes for poisons and a first aid booklet may also be kept with the medicines.

9. When the medicine is no longer needed, empty the bottle into the toilet or drain, because:

    a. Many medicines spoil with age.

    b. Some medicines grow stronger with age and are dangerous to use again.

    c. Some medicines weaken with age.

    d. The original purpose of the medicine may be forgotten or the label may not be easily read. Unlabeled medicine should always be destroyed.

10. Remember the "five rights" in giving medicine:

The right medicine.	In the right manner.
To the right patient.	In the right amount.
At the right time.	

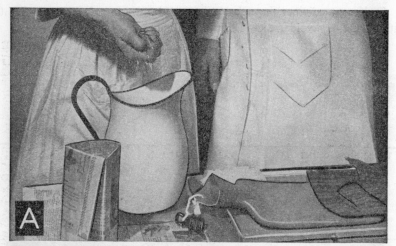

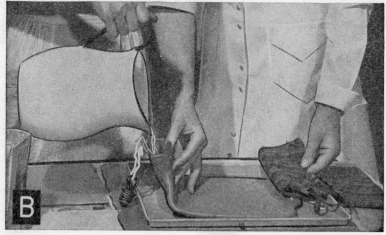

Preparing a hot water bag. (A) Test water with clenched fist. (B) Fill slowly, about half full.

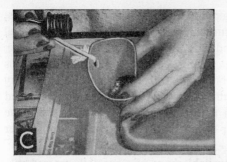

(C) Expel air from bag.
(D) Test for leaks.
(E) Cover.

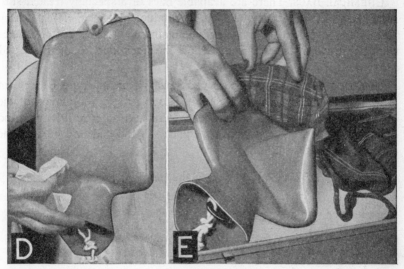

HOT APPLICATIONS

Purpose. Hot applications are used under certain conditions to relieve pain, increase the blood supply to an affected part of the body, give comfort, and promote healing.

Hot applications may take the form of dry or moist heat. Examples of dry heat are hot water bags, sun lamps or the sun itself, and electric pads. Moist heat may be in the form of a hot bath, foot bath, sitz bath or soak of any part of the body, or hot wet compresses. A steam inhalation and a hot throat irrigation are also forms of moist heat.

Hot Dry Applications.

HOT WATER BAG. A rubber hot water bag is commonly used to apply dry heat. Many substitutes may be used for a hot water bag, such as a brick, an iron, a plate, or a bag of sand or salt heated in the oven. Because it is more difficult to regulate the degree of heat of such substitutes, all should be adequately and securely wrapped. A crock or glass jar full of hot water, securely sealed and carefully protected against breakage, may also serve as a substitute. A connected electric iron is too dangerous to use. Woolen blankets heated on a radiator or in front of a stove may be used to provide added warmth, especially for babies; these covered with another blanket will retain the heat for quite a while. The home nurse should test the heat on her own skin; if comfortably warm for her it will be safe and effective for a baby.

CHEMICAL BAGS. There are available bags of a specially treated substance to which water may be added to produce heat by chemical action. These are convenient for travel and maintain an even heat but are somewhat expensive in the long run. Follow the directions for their use and care.

ELECTRIC PADS. Keep electric pads away from moisture because of the possible danger of a short circuit. Provide close observation of the patient, especially if an electric pad is to remain on over a long period of time; follow the directions that come with the pad and be sure the cord is in good condition.

Filling and Applying the Hot Water Bag
Equipment

Hot water bag with a stopper, washer, and cover
Container—preferably a pitcher
Supply of hot water
Supply of cold water
Cloth or paper wipes
Waste container

Procedure

1. Mix the water in a container and test; it should be momentarily bearable to a clenched fist thrust into the hot water, or approximately 115° to 130° F.

2. Fill the bag one-third to one-half full—so that the bag will be lightweight.

3. Expel the air—to make the bag pliable—place the bag on a flat surface and press until the water appears in the neck; screw in the stopper in this position.

4. Dry the bag and the inside of the neck. Test for leakage by holding upside down.

5. Put on the cover (of soft material).

6. Place with the hard neck of the bag away from the patient—for comfort.

7. Remove when cool; refill as needed.

8. Care for the bag after use. Allow the bag to drain dry; allow air to enter and screw in the stopper to keep the sides from sticking; put away in a dry, cool place. Put the cover in the laundry.

9. Note on the daily record where the bag was applied, for how long, and the reaction of the patient.

Hot Moist Applications (Compresses).

Woolen, gauze, or other soft material may be used for hot moist applications or compresses.

Hot applications may be large or small, depending upon the surface to be covered. They should be only large enough to cover the affected part completely. The doctor will order a special solution if plain water is not adequate. A wringer is suggested for a large compress. (*See* Making Substitute Equipment, p. 202.)

Applying a Hot Moist Compress, Using a Wringer
Equipment

1 or 2 basins
2 compresses of wool or soft cotton material, large enough to cover the affected area
Waxed paper to cover the compress
Piece of dry woolen cloth to cover the waxed paper and compress
Binder—a strip of cloth or a towel to be pinned over the compress to hold it in place
Safety pins
Bed cradle (*see* p. 207) if the bedclothes must be held away from the affected area

Kettle of boiling water
Wringer with a rod through the hem at both ends (*see* p. 216)—a bath towel or when large areas of the body are to be covered and strips of blanket are used as a compress, a wash wringer will be more practical
Protection for the table
Medication, if ordered

Procedure

1. Adjust the patient comfortably. Place the binder in position and have a dry woolen cloth, waxed paper, and safety pins handy at the bedside. Protect the table.

2. Arrange the wringer in the basin with the rod ends hanging over the sides. Place the folded compress within the folds of the wringer.

3. Pour enough boiling water over the compress to saturate it.

4. Wring dry—turn the rods in opposite directions; twist and pull to avoid knotting the wringer.

5. Empty the water from the basin; replace the wringer (with compress) covered with a second basin, if available, to keep the compress hot; and take to the bedside.

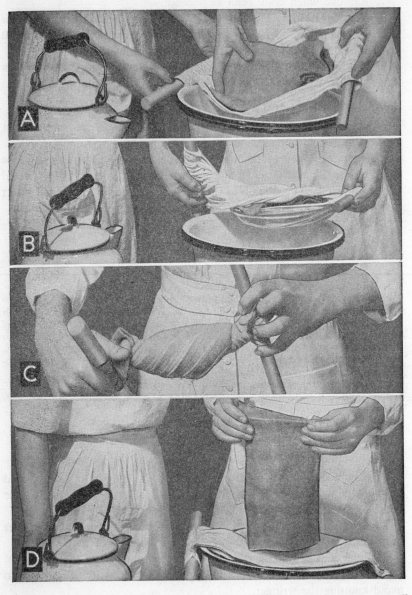

How to prepare a hot moist dressing. (A) Place flannel dressing in "wringer" and pour boiling water over it (B) Turn ends of wringer in opposite directions. (C) Wring dry. (D) Shake with quick movement to remove steam.

6. Expose the area where the compress is to be applied.

7. Remove the hot compress from the wringer; give two quick shakes to unfold and *remove the steam*—apply gradually to the patient's skin.

8. Cover the compress with waxed paper, then with a dry woolen cloth to keep in the heat.

9. Adjust the binder and pin securely.

10. A hot water bag may be used to help keep the compress hot.

11. Arrange a cradle to keep the bedclothes off the affected part, if needed.

12. Adjust the posture to be sure the patient is relaxed and comfortable.

13. Replace the compress as needed—about every 20 minutes—and continue the heat as long as ordered.

14. To discontinue treatment:
   a. Remove the wet compress. Make sure the patient is dry and warm. Leave the dry woolen cloth on the affected part for a brief period to avoid sudden chilling.
   b. Clear away the equipment; let the wringer and compresses dry.

15. Note on the daily record the time treatment was started and discontinued and any unusual appearance of the skin, comment made by the patient, or results of treatment observed.

Essential Points To Remember.

1. Obtain advice from the doctor before applying heat for a pain in the abdomen or stomach. The pain may be nature's warning of trouble, such as an inflamed appendix, for which heat may be the worst possible treatment.

2. Use great care to avoid burning when applying heat to the skin, especially of a person who is unconscious, paralyzed, very young, very old, a diabetic, or has edema (puffiness of the skin).

3. Use care when the skin is exposed to the rays of the sun. Excessive exposure may not only be painful but may result in serious harm to the body. Do not give a sun bath to a baby without instructions from the doctor.

4. Use a sun lamp on the doctor's order only and follow exactly the directions that come with the lamp. Do not let a patient fall asleep under a sun lamp.

5. When filling the hot water bag:
   a. Prepare the water in a container to allow testing the temperature —"momentarily bearable to the clenched fist."
   b. Watch for leaks.

6. When applying hot moist compress:
   a. Wring out the excess water.
   b. Shake out the steam.
   c. Keep the compress hot enough to be effective and yet not burn.

COLD APPLICATIONS

Purpose. Cold is often applied to relieve pain and congestion.

Cold applied to the skin contracts the blood vessels near the surface, relieving pain due to swelling and congestion. Used for brief periods at a time, cold has a stimulating effect on circulation and muscle tissue. Cold applications are not frequently used for people who are in a weakened condition. Cold applications may be either dry or moist.

Dry Cold Applications

An ice cap, ice collar, or substitute is usually used. Some possible substitutes are a hot water bag filled with finely crushed ice or ice water, or a rubber swimming cap filled with crushed ice and tied securely.

Filling and Applying an Ice Bag

Equipment

Rubber ice bag with a cap,   Container of finely cracked ice
washer, and cover

Procedure

1. Fill the ice bag about one-half full.
2. To expel the air from the bag, squeeze the bag so ice appears in the neck.
3. Screw on the top—be sure the washer is in place.
4. Dry the bag and put on the cover.
5. Apply to the affected part and watch for leaks.
6. Renew ice as needed.
7. Discontinue treatment as ordered, and note the patient's reaction on the daily record.
8. Care for the equipment:
   a. Empty and dry the bag—inflate it with air. Screw on the cap and put away in a dry, cool place.
   b. Put the cover in the laundry.

Moist Cold Applications

Equipment

Compresses the size of the area to be   Basin of pieces of ice
covered and moistened with water

Procedure

1. Place the patient in a comfortable position and provide protection.
2. Place the moistened compress on ice to cool.
3. Wring the compress free of dripping water and apply to the affected area (leave uncovered).
4. Place another compress on the ice to cool.
5. Change the compresses as needed (about every 3 minutes).
6. Discontinue the treatment as ordered and note the patient's reaction on the daily record.
7. Care of equipment:
   a. Empty the basin and cleanse thoroughly.
   b. Discard the compresses.

Essential Points To Remember.

1. Avoid too long exposure to cold. Watch for chilling and a bluish color of the skin.
2. Watch for leaks in ice bags.
3. When applying moist cold applications, avoid using finely crushed ice, which tends to adhere to the compress and cause discomfort.

INSPECTING THE THROAT

Purpose. To see if there is marked redness or swelling or visible spots or patches on the throat and to be able to describe to the doctor the condition observed.

When the throat is being inspected, it is also well to note the condition of the tongue, gums, and teeth and the odor of the breath. To

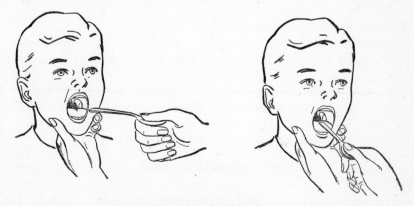

Inspecting the throat.

gain the coöperation of a child, it is wise to practice this procedure when he is well.

Equipment

A clean teaspoon   Perhaps a flashlight

Procedure

1. Explain to the patient what is to be done.
2. Place the patient where the light is good—near a window or lamp —or use a flashlight.
3. Steady the patient's chin with one hand.
4. Ask him to open his mouth wide and say "Ah." This relaxes the throat for a better view.
5. Place the *handle* of a teaspoon about two-thirds back on the tongue.
6. Press down very gently so that the back of the throat is in clear view. Ask the patient to say "Ah" again.
7. Inspect the back and sides of the throat for redness, swelling, and white, gray, or yellowish patches. If unable to observe well on the first attempt, let the patient rest and inspect again. Avoid touching the soiled part of the spoon until it has been properly washed.

What To Report to the Doctor

If there are white, gray, or yellowish patches in the throat or if the throat is unusually red or swollen, take the patient's temperature; report the conditions to the doctor; put the patient to bed and keep him and the things he uses away from others.

Essential Points To Remember.

1. Avoid making the patient gag.
2. Avoid direct contact with the nose or throat spray in case the patient coughs.
3. Deposit the spoon directly in a container for proper cleansing.
4. Keep any person with a sore throat away from others.

INHALATIONS AND THROAT IRRIGATIONS

Purpose. To relieve hoarseness, sore throat, coughing, or difficulty in breathing.

Heat is sometimes ordered in the form of a steam inhalation. The patient breathes—inhales—the steam from heated water, thus bringing heat directly to the tissues of the nose, throat, and bronchial tubes, which may be swollen and painful as a result of infection. Medicines that vaporize are sometimes ordered so that the steam carries their vapor to the tissues.

Giving a Steam Inhalation to a Patient in Bed

Equipment

Teakettle or other container of boiling water—or a commercial inhalator
Protected chair, stool, or box for the kettle or container
Medication, if ordered, placed in a can or other small container (weighted to prevent spilling)
Extra pillow

Extra shawl or blanket, if needed
Paper tissues
Paper cornucopia or funnel—a long tube
Towel to cover the hair
Umbrella or other tent frame
Blanket or other means of making a tent cover

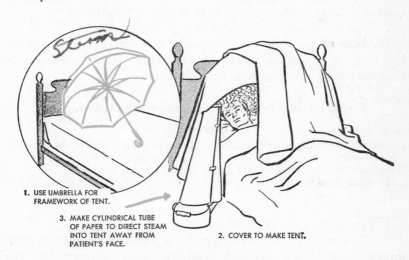

1. USE UMBRELLA FOR FRAMEWORK OF TENT.

3. MAKE CYLINDRICAL TUBE OF PAPER TO DIRECT STEAM INTO TENT AWAY FROM PATIENT'S FACE.

2. COVER TO MAKE TENT.

Improvising a steam tent.

Procedure

1. Assemble the equipment; arrange the patient comfortably in bed; protect the working areas.

2. Measure the medication, if ordered, into the weighted can and place in the kettle—with the water level lower than the top of the can. Prevent the medicine from staining the inside of the kettle.

3. Support the patient's head with the extra pillow; place the extra covering over his shoulders; protect his hair with a towel and provide tissues to wipe the patient's face.

4. Make a tent—adjust the opened umbrella or frame over the patient's head and shoulders; cover well with the blanket; leave an open air space in front.

5. Place the kettle with the steaming water on a protected surface at the bedside and fit one end of the funnel over the spout and open top of the kettle and the other end under the tent. Keep the kettle out of reach of the patient.

6. Direct the steam toward the top of the tent and away from the patient's face.

7. Maintain steam in the kettle by changing the water when necessary. Remain near at hand to give assistance if needed.

8. Discontinue the inhalation at the time indicated; remove the equipment; dry the patient's face; prevent chilling. The patient should remain quiet in a warm room for about an hour after the treatment.

9. Care for the equipment after use: Put away clean.

10. Note on the daily record the time treatment was given and for how long, the patient's comments, and any improvement noted, such as easier breathing, less coughing, or less hoarseness.

Giving a Steam Inhalation to a Patient Who Is Sitting Up

Equipment

Container of steaming water (a pitcher is convenient)

Paper sack with a "window" cut for the steam to escape

Basin in which to place the container (for safety)

Towel to cover the hair

Procedure

1. Protect the hair and shoulders.

2. The container with steaming water is placed in a basin at a comfortable height; the paper sack is inverted over the container. The patient leans forward and breathes in warm, moist air through the hole in the paper sack.

Giving Inhalations to Babies and Little Children

Babies and children suffering from bronchitis, laryngitis, colds, croup, or asthma often benefit greatly from breathing in warmed moist air. To moisten the air of the room it is usually sufficient to have a kettle or vaporizer filled with water kept boiling at some safe spot in the room at a distance from the bed. Sometimes the doctor orders a "croup tent." Arrange a tent or canopy over the child's crib and direct the steam from the vaporizer or kettle so it will flow into the tent, keeping it away from the child's face. The treatment is generally ordered for 20 or 30 minutes but may be ordered for much longer. The doctor will say what medicine he wishes used for the vaporizer, if any.

If the child is old enough, explain what is to be done; little children like the tent if it is treated as part of a game and they may sit up or lie down in the tent.

As a safety measure always stay with a child who is in a croup tent! Be sure that the vaporizer or kettle is placed safely out of reach of the child and that the steam is kept up as needed.

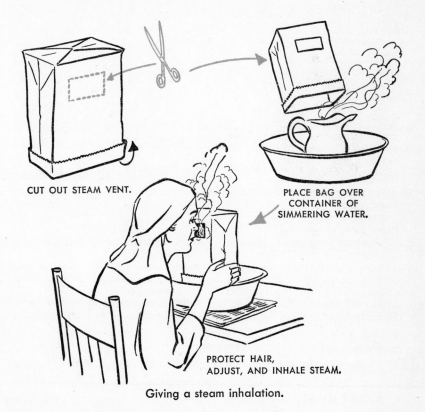

CUT OUT STEAM VENT.

PLACE BAG OVER
CONTAINER OF
SIMMERING WATER.

PROTECT HAIR,
ADJUST, AND INHALE STEAM.

Giving a steam inhalation.

Essential Points To Remember.

1. Avoid burning the patient with steam—direct the steam away from the patient's skin.

2. Avoid fire when using an electric device—keep the device away from the bedding or remain in the room continuously.

3. Provide adequate steam for effective results.

4. Make the patient comfortable during treatment.

5. Avoid chilling the patient after treatment.

Throat Irrigation

Purpose. To relieve pain, redness, swelling, and tightness in the throat by applying hot moist heat directly to the tissues (mucous membranes) that line the throat.

A throat irrigation is a way of applying moist heat directly to the tissues (mucous membranes) that line the throat. It is used when infection or inflammation is present and is usually ordered several times a day. Salt is sometimes added to the water, 2 teaspoonfuls to 1 quart. A throat irrigation should be given only when ordered by the doctor, as there are some types of sore throat in which the application of heat might do harm. If able, the patient may sit up in bed or beside the bowl or the toilet in the bathroom. If lying or sitting in bed, the head and shoulders should be well propped up, the head to the side or forward, so that water will not run down the throat; the room should be warm and free from drafts.

Little children, too young to understand how to take this treatment, should not be given throat irrigations.

Equipment

Clean fountain syringe or irrigating can with tubing

Clean connecting tubing with a blunt end that cannot injure the throat— a hard rubber nozzle or soft rubber tubing (boil the part that goes into the mouth)

Waste container (pail, toilet bowl) for the return flow

Rubber apron, rubber sheet, or several newspapers and a large towel for protection

Solution as ordered by the doctor

Cold cream or oil to protect the skin

Procedure

1. Explain to the patient what is going to be done and how he can assist.

2. Protect the bed and patient.

3. Protect the chin with cold cream or oil.

4. Adjust the irrigating can; the water solution should be 4 to 6 inches higher than the patient's head to insure a gentle rate of flow. Regulate the flow by raising or lowering the can or closing the tubing.

5. Test the water—it should be hot enough to produce a slight sting to the wrist.

Red Cross

HOME

NURSING

Civil Defense Supplement

*for Red Cross
Home Nurses
and Volunteer
Nurse's Aides*

The American National Red Cross

WASHINGTON, D. C.

ARC 1644
JANUARY 1951

INTRODUCTION

The world was shocked in 1945 by the thousands killed at Hiroshima and Nagaski by atom bombs. However, the number of dead and injured could have been greatly lessened if the Japanese could have known what to expect and how to care for themselves.

Self-help is a fundamental factor in civil defense. This means that everyone must be willing and able to help himself and his neighbors. In a great emergency, those who have had appropriate training will have the best chance for survival—it is important that everyone be prepared to care for himself and others.

Not only must great reliance be placed upon self-help within families, but blocks, neighborhoods, and communities must be ready to meet the needs of thousands who may be injured or ill. Immediately following a bomb attack, you may be sharing your house with strangers or you may be one of many people in a shelter where only the necessities are available. People who have had some training will be able to give care to the sick or injured and to handle many routine, time-consuming duties for overtaxed nursing personnel.

Those who have had a home nursing course or a volunteer nurse's aide course will assume important roles as assistants to professional nurses in the event of a major catastrophe. Volunteer nurse's aides, because of their broader training and experience, will be expected to carry more responsibility than home nurses. Many who have taken these courses will be asked to accept assignments as nurse assistants in civil defense, and appropriate instructions will be given by local civil defense authorities.

Everyone who participates in civil defense activities should take a Red Cross first aid course.

In some situations the need for nursing care may extend over a prolonged period. Physicians or professional nurses will be responsible for the over-all care of these patients and will give specific directions concerning nursing care to the nurse assistants. During catastrophies, however, professional people may not always be immediately available, and nurse assistants may have to assume responsibilities that are far beyond those usually expected of them.

The nursing care required for injuries and illnesses resulting from a major disaster or modern warfare is similar to that needed in normal situations. But caring for a large number of patients under difficult conditions makes it necessary for a nurse assistant to have additional preparation. For example, certain symptoms will take on new importance in the event of modern warfare and the need to improvise equipment and supplies will be great.

In any emergency the behavior of individuals is unpredictable. Some respond with courage and immediately make themselves useful, while others are confused or frightened into helplessness. People trained in home nursing or as nurse's aides will be expected to give reassurance to family members and others in the neighborhood or community. Small

1

children who experience a calamity of any kind need the reassuring presence of family members to avoid additional emotional strain. For this reason, mothers should remain with their children whenever possible.

Major disasters and modern warfare not only cause extensive injuries, they also may expose persons in the affected areas to other dangers, such as:

1. Illness resulting from exposure and fatigue.

2. Infections caused by increased contamination of wounds.

3. Increased danger of spreading communicable diseases because of overcrowding and other unsanitary conditions.

Nurse's aides and home nurses can make an immediate contribution to civil defense by encouraging family members, especially children, and neighbors to become immunized against those diseases for which there is protection, such as diphtheria, whooping cough, and smallpox. Tetanus immunization should be emphasized as a protection in case of injury.

In modern warfare there is the possibility of the need for rapid evacuation of some hospital patients—the aged, the chronically ill, and the convalescent—to make room for serious cases in need of immediate hospitalization. The evacuees will require continuing care at home or in designated centers and will have to help themselves as much as possible. Under supervision, nurse's aides and home nurses will be expected to give routine care to these patients.

During an emergency the variety and kinds of food available may be limited, but as nourishment is always important for the sick and injured, nurse assistants will undoubtedly be called upon to help feed people as regularly and adequately as possible. The dangers of food-borne disease outbreaks and of food contaminated by radioactivity should be kept in mind; local civil defense authorities will issue special instructions to combat these problems if they arise.

SOME RESPONSIBILITIES OF HOME NURSES AND NURSE'S AIDES

Under emergency conditions home nurses and nurse's aides might be expected to perform the following duties in their own homes, in shelters, emergency hospitals, or emergency medical stations.

Provide Usual Nursing Care. During the immediate emergency period good general nursing care is of primary importance for all patients. For example, patients may be frightened, cold, hungry, or thirsty. Keep them quiet and make them comfortable as quickly as possible by providing proper support, covers, and whatever food and liquids are permitted and available. Continued nursing care will depend upon the needs of each patient and the directions of the doctor or nurse in charge.

Reassure Patients and Families. The nurse assistant who is calm and well informed about the condition of her patients can lighten the workload of doctors and nurses by reassuring patients and their families. It is of the utmost importance that patients and their families be assured that everything possible is being done to promote recovery. It is equally important that doctors and nurses be relieved of as much routine work as possible.

Report Unusual Symptoms of Injury or Illness. The limited number of professional nurses will make it necessary for nurse assistants to assume greater responsibility in recording and reporting symptoms observed while giving care. For symptoms of particular importance under wartime conditions, see pp. 6-10.

Help Set Up and Improvise Equipment and Supplies. Nurse assistants will help to assemble, improvise, and keep in order stocks of medical supplies and equipment wherever they may be needed. Limited facilities and supplies will necessitate many adaptations. For example, newspapers may be used under pallets or mattresses on the floor as a protection against moisture and cold; blankets or clothing may be rolled and used as pillows; drinking cups may be made from clean paper; tin cans, glass jars, paper cartons, or pans may be used for vomitus or as bedpans and urinals. (See "Making Substitute Equipment," *American Red Cross Home Nursing Textbook,* pp. 202-17.)

Handwashing facilities may be limited, but nurse assistants can still carry out the principles of cleanliness to protect patients and themselves from infection by:

1. Not touching body discharges.
2. Using newspapers to handle and dispose of material contaminated by body discharges.
3. Grasping a relatively clean area of soiled dressings.
4. Keeping their hands away from their own faces.

Observe Patients Receiving Intravenous Injections. When patients are being given plasma, whole blood, or other fluids, it is important to follow instructions carefully:

1. Be sure the needle stays in place. Keep patient quiet, especially that part of body where needle is inserted.
2. Watch the container and report if fluid stops flowing.
3. Watch for and report any swelling around needle.
4. Watch for and report immediately any signs of the patient's being chilly or shivering.
5. Remain with patient until doctor or nurse arrives.

Stay with Patient Coming Out of an Anesthetic. Because of her training and experience in hospitals, a volunteer nurse's aide will usually be given this assignment. It is important to follow instructions carefully:

1. Keep patient quiet and warm.

2. Give fluids only as ordered and never to unconscious patient.

3. Watch for vomiting; provide a container.

4. Keep patient's head turned to the side so that fluid will run out of his mouth easily.

5. Take and record pulse rate frequently during the first 24 hours. Report any significant change to doctor or nurse.

6. Watch for signs of bleeding on the dressings and report.

7. Watch for swelling of the abdomen and report.

8. Note the color of the skin—paleness or blueness may indicate shock; report to doctor or nurse.

9. Watch for breathing difficulties; if present push lower jaw forward by pressure on the angle of the jaw just below the tip of the ear and call for assistance.

Assist with Special Treatments Under Supervision. Nurse assistants may help to apply dressings, bearing in mind the principles of cleanliness as emphasized in the nurse's aide and home nursing courses. In addition, nurse assistants will be given instructions regarding their responsibilities when assisting with special treatments. As a part of the civil defense plans of a local community, standardized treatments for specific conditions, such as burns, may be set up by the local medical group. In any event, general directions for the patient's care between visits of the physician or nurse will be available in each situation.

Help Give Nourishment to Patients. (See textbook, chapter 4.) Modifications in feeding may be made in accordance with the number and needs of patients and availability of food. The nurse assistant will be given instructions by a doctor or nurse in making these modifications. In burn cases, for example, the doctor may order a high protein diet. Many patients will need assistance while eating, and the nurse assistant should observe the needs of each patient and give help accordingly.

Food or liquids should not be given by mouth if a patient is unconscious, is unable to swallow, faces early surgery, or has an abdominal injury.

For some patients the doctor will order the amount of liquids to be given and will request measurement of the liquids taken.

Protect Patients from Additional Hazards. To avoid further injury or unnecessary discomfort, a nurse assistant should be aware of hazardous conditions, such as loose plaster, shattered glass, gas leaks, leaking roofs, wet floors, and possible fires. These conditions should be reported to the person in charge immediately.

Prepare Patients for Transfer. Patients may be sent out of emergency centers within the first day or two—either to hospitals or to other centers for further care. It may be the nurse assistant's responsibility to prepare these patients for transfer. Essential points to remember are:

1. Reassure the patient.
2. Make the patient as comfortable as possible on the carrying vehicle, with body in proper position and with support for injured part.
3. Be sure litter bearer or other person has been given special orders regarding the position of injured parts and, if necessary, show how to place and maintain the needed support.
4. If there are extensive wounds, be sure they are securely bandaged.
5. Check to be sure that a copy of the patient's medical record accompanies him and that the last medication or nursing care given is recorded.
6. If the transfer is to be over some distance or if delay is likely, see that a drink or nourishment is given, if permitted, and offer bedpan or urinal.
7. Selected personal belongings should be tied together and sent with the patient, if practical.

INJURIES AND ILLNESSES FREQUENTLY ENCOUNTERED IN EMERGENCY SITUATIONS

When disaster strikes, either natural or man-made, the injuries and illnesses most frequently encountered that require nursing care are:

1. Open cuts and other wounds from glass and debris.
2. Fractures.
3. Bruises.
4. Pressure or crushing injuries.
5. Concussion.
6. Hemorrhage—internal and external.
7. Burns from heat, fire, steam, or hot water.
8. Shock—immediate and delayed.
9. Illnesses resulting from fatigue, exposure, and overcrowding, often under unsanitary conditions. The very young or the aged will be particularly affected.
10. Childbirth, premature or at term, or abortion may be expected.

In addition, under conditions of atomic warfare, there will be radiation sickness—caused by the rays liberated by an atom bomb. There may be other special types of warfare, such as chemical or bacteriological. Advice with regard to these will be given through the local civil defense group when necessary.

GUIDE FOR NURSE ASSISTANTS

CONDITION	WHAT TO OBSERVE	WHAT TO DO	WHAT TO REPORT

1. Shock
 	
Failure of circulation. Every injured person may be in shock and should be regarded as such until diagnosis is made.
Evidence of shock may be delayed.
	Weakness and faintness.
	Dizziness and nausea.
	Skin pale, cold with perspiration.
	Eyes vacant and lackluster.
	Rapid heartbeat and therefore rapid pulse.
	Air hunger — breathing shallow and rapid with later, irregular, sighing respirations.
	Excessive thirst.
	Signs of external or internal hemorrhage.
		Notify doctor at once.
		Conserve body heat but do not overheat; keep patient on the edge of chilliness.
		Later may need to apply external heat.
		Tilt patient so that blood tends to flow to upper portions of the body. Head and chest should be about 6-12 inches lower than the rest of the body.
		Give other care as ordered.
			Symptoms of shock:
			  Air hunger.
			  Rapid pulse, growing weaker.
			  Excessive thirst, mouth dry.

2. Cuts and Wounds	Location of cuts and jagged wounds. Bleeding. Glass or other debris in wound. Symptoms of shock or signs of internal bleeding that resemble shock (some puncture wounds may be deeper than first suspected). Evidence of pain. Discharge, amount and odor. Swelling. Discoloration, red streaks leading away from wound.	Keep wound clean and covered—apply sterile dressing. Support affected part and, if sensitive, prevent weight of bedclothes. If bleeding shows through dressing, apply fresh dressing over original dressing, using slight pressure. Later, doctor may order movement of affected part to help prevent stiffening of joints.	Symptoms of shock or internal bleeding. Changes in color, odor, or consistency of discharge from wound. Swelling about the wound. Red streaks leading away from wound. Evidence of foreign object in wound.

6

3. Hemorrhage	External:
	  Force—dripping, spurting.
	  Amount.
	  Color; bright or dark red.
	  Location.
	Internal:
	  Air hunger—gasping or deep sighing.
	  Rapid pulse, growing weaker.
	  Sense of smothering.
	  Excessive thirst, mouth dry.
	  Restlessness.
	  Skin cold, clammy, pale, or bluish.
	  Apparent source, such as lung (frothy), rectum, or other.
		Notify doctor or nurse at once.
		Reassure patient; keep him quiet.
		Keep patient comfortably warm.
		Supply fluids *unless otherwise ordered.* Begin with about 1 cupful every hour if tolerated. (No stimulants.)
		If external:
		  Apply sterile dressing and bandage; apply pressure over the dressing to help control bleeding.
		If internal:
		  See textbook, pp. 90–91.
			Air hunger.
			Rapid pulse.
			Excessive thirst.
			Fall in temperature.
			Skin: cold, clammy, pale, or blue.
			Continued bleeding.

4. Burns	Reddened skin, accompanied by pain—first degree. Blisters with some pain—second degree. Cooking or charring, usually little pain except around edges of wound—third degree. Extent of burns: Particularly dangerous if large areas of body surface involved, such as face, arm, back, or chest, in which case shock is likely to develop. Evidence of infection.	Treat for shock. Leave face unbandaged. Expose wound, removing only large, easily separated foreign particles, such as clothing or debris. Apply thick, dry, sterile dressing; avoid wrinkling and overlapping. Apply separate dressings to each finger or toe. Bandage firmly. Give medication as ordered by doctor. Keep patient comfortably warm. Give general nursing care, keeping body in position to help prevent deformity. Give fluids—about 1 cupful every hour unless otherwise ordered. Measure and record fluid intake and urine output.	Symptoms of shock. Any sudden rise in temperature, which may indicate infection. Change in urinary output—amount, color, odor, or evidence of sediment.

CONDITION	WHAT TO OBSERVE	WHAT TO DO	WHAT TO REPORT
5. Fractures— Simple and Compound	Pain upon motion or tenderness of injured part. Inability to use injured part. Patient sometimes moves part below break. Deformity (meaning out of normal shape) sometimes detectable. External wound—bone may protrude in compound fracture. Swelling, blueness, or numbness of toes or fingers if in cast or bandaged. Complaint of pressure or pain under cast or bandage. Evidence of loose cast or bandage. Evidence of pressure sores.	Keep injured part in good position at all times. Get plenty of help when moving patient to avoid further injury. Provide support for correct position and for comfort, such as pads, pillows, etc. (See textbook, chapter 9.) If patient is in traction, keep traction taut (without slack) at all times. Keep skin clean, dry, and free from pressure. (See textbook, chapter 9.)	Any unusual swelling around bandage or cast; any blueness, swelling, or numbness of protruding parts, such as toes, or complaint of undue pressure at any particular point. An injured part moving too freely within bandage or cast. Any indication of pressure sores or reddened areas on skin over bony prominences. Inability to move any part of body.
6. Severe Bruises and Crushing Injuries	Discolored areas of skin—black, blue, red. Flattened or mashed extremities, with accompanying bleeding. Evidence of pain. Difficulty in breathing if chest injury. Discharge. Break in skin.	Give general nursing care. Elevate and support injured part in correct position. Apply heat or cold only when instructed to do so. Treat any break in the skin as an open wound. If chest injury, causing breathing difficulty, keep air passages open by turning head to one side to allow fluid to run out.	Discharges from or change in color and texture of injured part. Change in color or amount of urine. Symptoms of shock. Change or difficulty in breathing.

8

Condition	Signs and Symptoms	Care	Report to Physician
7. Concussion and Other Head Injuries	Complaint of headache. Period of unconsciousness. Unusual behavior—may be excitable or stuporous. Heavy breathing. Bleeding or discharge. Vomiting, especially when forceful. Swelling or lump on head. Face flushed or pale. Evidence of dizziness, pain, or convulsions.	Keep patient lying down. Provide warmth. Apply sterile dressing to any wound. Avoid giving fluids until ordered by the doctor. Avoid giving alcoholic beverage or stimulants, such as coffee, tea, or cocoa. Avoid swabbing inside ears or nose if there is bleeding. Count pulse frequently during the first 24 hours to note any change in rate or condition. Measure fluids given and output of urine. If breathing is difficult, keep air passages open by turning head to one side to allow fluid to run out and, if necessary, push lower jaw forward by pressing on the angle of the jaw just below tip of ear.	Bleeding: indicate source, such as from ears, nose, or open scalp wound. Rise in temperature. Sudden change in pulse rate. Forceful vomiting—explosive. Symptoms of shock. Deep unconsciousness.
8. Reaction from Intravenous Injections Plasma. Whole blood. Other fluids.	Swelling around point of injection. Complaint of chilliness. Real chill—shivering, chattering teeth, and convulsive movements of body.	Obtain help from doctor or nurse *immediately.* Be reassuring.	Report immediately any swelling around point of injection, complaint of chilliness or noticeable shivering, if solution in the container ceases to flow, or if needle comes out.
9. Radiation Sickness	Nausea and vomiting. Diarrhea—blood in stool. Weakness and headache. Evidence of sore throat.	Keep patient away from others who have a communicable disease, such as a cold.	Signs of shock. Nausea and vomiting.

GUIDE FOR NURSE ASSISTANTS (Continued)

CONDITION	WHAT TO OBSERVE	WHAT TO DO	WHAT TO REPORT
9. Radiation Sickness (*Continued*)	Tiny hemorrhages (discolorations) in the skin, which gradually become larger and break open. Bleeding from gums and other mucous membrane. Symptoms may occur the first day but often may be delayed for a week or more. Location of patient at time of bomb burst important in diagnosis.	Keep all wounds clean and covered with sterile dressings. Keep patient as quiet as possible. Give general nursing care.	Bleeding from gums or other mucous membrane. Enlarging bruiselike areas on skin. Bloody diarrhea. Evidence of sore throat. Rise in temperature.

ESSENTIAL POINTS TO REMEMBER

1. The need for professional guidance—where and how to obtain it. 2. The value of practicing skills to develop confidence. 3. The importance of keeping calm and giving assistance in time of crisis.

Skill inspires self-confidence; a well-grounded faith in one's own ability is a primary requisite for service to others; training and preparation build security for yourself, your family, your community, and the nation.

6. Instruct the patient to breathe through his nose and let the hot solution flow in one side of the mouth, over the throat, and out the other side of the mouth. If able, the patient may hold the irrigating tip and direct the flow. Irrigate first one side of the throat, then the other. Be sure to direct the flow at the side of the throat to avoid gagging. The flow should be smooth and steady. The patient may hold a basin under his chin to receive the return flow. Tell the patient to avoid swallowing the solution, although it will do no harm if a little rolls down his throat.

7. After completing the treatment, dry the face gently; remove the protecting covers and make the patient comfortable; avoid chilling.

8. Care of the equipment after use:

    a. Wash the bag or can and tubing with hot soapy water; rinse with clear water and allow to drain dry.

    b. Put away the fountain syringe or tubing in a cool dry place; avoid bending or folding the tubing—it may crack.

    c. Empty the waste basin or pail and scrub with hot soapy water; rinse with scalding water and allow to dry.

    d. Scrub the irrigating tip or nozzle with hot soapy water; rinse and then boil for 5 minutes. Allow to dry. Keep with the equipment.

9. Note on the daily record the time the irrigation was given and amount, the appearance of the return flow, and the patient's reaction and condition as observed.

Essential Points To Remember.

1. Avoid burning the patient—the water should be hot enough to be effective but not hot enough to burn.

2. Irrigate the throat only when ordered by the doctor.

3. Thoroughly cleanse the equipment before and after use.

STERILE DRESSINGS

A sterile dressing is one free from disease germs. When there is a break in the skin, the dressing should be sterile.

Dry Sterile Dressings

Purpose. To protect a wound and absorb any discharge.

Equipment

Package of sterile dressings
Bandage (roller or triangular)
Strips of adhesive tape or safety pins
Scissors

Knife or spoon
Medication, if ordered
Waste container
Support for the part to be dressed

Procedure

1. Place the patient in a sitting or lying down position. Support the part to be dressed.

2. Assemble the materials; leave the sterile package unopened. Cut the desired length of adhesive strip or strips.

3. Wash the hands thoroughly, using soap and water; rinse; shake off water.

4. Expose the affected area. When the soiled dressing is removed, handle only at the extreme edge and drop into the waste container for disposal.

5. Open the dressing package, touching only the edges. Unfold, if necessary. Place the inside surface of the dressing next to the wound.

6. If ointment is ordered, squeeze it from the tube onto the dressing and spread by folding the dressing together. Open out the dressing and apply. If the ointment is in a jar, spread it on the dressing with a knife or spoon that has been boiled. *Spread the ointment on the dressing rather than directly on the wound.*

7. Make the dressing secure with adhesive, or bandage, or both.

8. Burn the soiled dressing if possible.

9. Put away the equipment.

10. Wash the hands thoroughly.

11. Note on the daily record the appearance of the wound and the condition of the patient.

Wet Sterile Dressings—Cold

Purpose. To keep a wound continuously moist, usually with some special solution and to promote drainage and healing.

Equipment

Package of sterile gauze dressings (several will be needed, as dry dressings are often used over the wet layer)
Waxed paper
Bandage or binder
Safety pins
Piece of dry flannel or other cloth for protection

Solution as ordered by the doctor
Sterile container and a cover for the solution
Lifter, such as tongs or forceps, if available, for handling the sterile dressings

Procedure

1. Place the patient in a comfortable position.

2. Assemble the equipment and protect the bed or area where the dressing is to be done. If tongs are used, they should be boiled, the water drained off, and the tongs left in a covered basin until used.

3. Loosen a package of sterile gauze dressings.

4. Uncover the solution. Be sure it is the proper temperature.

5. Fold back the bedclothes; remove all but one soiled dressing and place in waste container. Leave one layer covering the affected area.

6. Explain to the patient that the hands must be washed again before the sterile dressing is handled. (This will not be necessary if tongs are used to handle the dressing.) Instruct the patient to keep his hands off the dressings and wound.

7. Wash the hands thoroughly, using friction; rinse; shake off water. (Omit this step if using tongs.)

8. Return to the bedside and remove the last layer, holding the dressing by a corner. (If the patient is able and wants to, he, instead of the home nurse, may lift this dressing and drop it in a waste container.)

9. Taking out the sterile dressing by a corner or with the tongs moisten in the sterile solution and apply. Before applying waxed paper, cover the wet dressing with two or three dry sterile dressings.

10. Secure with a bandage or binder.

11. Wash the hands thoroughly. If the patient has touched the soiled dressings, he must wash his hands also.

12. Keep the dressing wet or moist by loosening the binder, cover, and waxed paper and gently pouring a little of the solution over it.

Wet Sterile Dressings—Hot

A *sterile* hot moist dressing is sometimes ordered by the doctor. Gauze or soft linen is usually used for a hot sterile dressing. Boiling is a simple way to prepare such a dressing in the home.

Equipment

See equipment for a wet sterile dressing.

Procedure

Proceed in the same way as for applying a hot moist compress (p. 183) with the following exceptions:

1. Boil the dressing and wringer before applying; also boil a pair of tongs or forceps (if available).

2. Handle the sterile dressing with the tongs, or, if by hand, touch only at the corners.

3. In removing the dressing from the affected area, if it is soiled with discharges, handle with care to avoid touching the soiled area. Dispose of the dressing in a waste container and burn, if possible.

Essential Points To Remember.

1. Use a dressing large enough to cover the wound completely and anchor it securely by using adhesive, a bandage, or both. Avoid the use of absorbent cotton, adhesive, collodion, or a similar preparation directly on a wound, as it might prevent healing, be difficult to remove, and cause pain.

2. Secure a dressing lightly but firmly. A tight bandage tends to interfere with the circulation, causing swelling. When a hand, arm, foot, or leg is bandaged, watch the nails; if they look bluish or if the patient complains of numbness, loosen the bandage.

3. Secure a wet bandage less firmly than a dry one. It will shrink as it dries and may become too tight. If the above symptoms are noted, loosen.

4. Antiseptic, if ordered for breaks in the skin, must be kept away from the eyes, mouth, or other body openings. Apply antiseptics with an applicator (cotton swab).

5. Always wash the hands before and after caring for a wound.

6. Report to the doctor:
   a. The condition of the wound being dressed: its appearance—discharge and amount, blood and amount, or healing.
   b. The patient's general condition.
   c. If wet dressings are being applied, the length of time applied and the appearance of the wound or skin afterward.

7. When applying a *hot* wet dressing:
   a. Wring out the excess water.
   b. Shake out the steam.
   c. Keep the dressing hot enough to be effective and yet not burn.

8. Wounds are subject to two dangers of special importance—*bleeding* (hemorrhage) and *infection*. In case of hemorrhage, apply pressure with a sterile compress and firm bandage; keep the patient quiet with the part elevated. If the hemorrhage cannot be controlled by applying pressure, send for the doctor at once. Look for signs of infection. These are swelling, redness, and, usually, pain. Later signs of infection are a discharge, fever, enlarged glands near the wound, and a general feeling of fatigue and sickness. Sometimes red streaks appear along the veins leading from the wound. Medical attention should be obtained as soon as any sign of infection is noted.

PUTTING DROPS IN THE EYES

Purpose. To relieve eye conditions, dilate the pupils for an oculist's examination, or soothe irritation. *Do this only when ordered by a doctor or oculist.*

Equipment

Drops *as prescribed by a doctor or oculist*
Clean medicine dropper attached to a bottle or separate

Paper tissues or wipes
Towel or other shoulder protection

Procedure

1. Ask the patient to sit on a chair facing a good light. The nurse should stand.

2. Protect the patient's shoulders.

3. Supply tissue with which to wipe the cheeks (not the eyes).

4. Check the label of the bottle.

5. *If a medicine dropper is attached to the bottle of eye drops,* draw up enough drops for both eyes as ordered, or *if the medicine dropper is separate,* uncork the bottle of eye drops (check the label) and place the cork upside down on the table. Draw up enough drops for both eyes as ordered.

6. Recheck the label on the bottle.

7. With the dropper in one hand, take the tissue in the other and gently draw down the under lid of the eye with the first two fingers resting on the tissue.

8. Ask the patient to look up and roll his eye without moving his head.

9. Holding the dropper above the lower lid *but not touching* the eye, lid, or lashes with the dropper, gently press out the number of drops ordered by the doctor, letting them fall in the lining of the *lower lid,* rather than on the eye.

10. Instruct the patient to close his eye gently and wipe his cheeks (but not his eye) if the drops run down.

11. Repeat at once if ordered for the other eye, not allowing the dropper to touch anything. Return the dropper to the bottle if there is a delay before treating the second eye—to keep the dropper and drops absolutely clean.

12. After both eyes are treated, return the dropper to the bottle. If using a separate dropper, rinse it thoroughly and put it away.

13. Instruct the patient not to rub his eyes.

14. Report on the daily record for the doctor the time the drops were administered, the condition of the eyes, and the patient's reaction then or later, if any.

Essential Points To Remember.

1. Keep the medicine dropper clean.
2. Handle the eyes gently.

3. Allow the medicine to drop on the lining of the lower lid.
4. Instruct the patient to keep his hands away from his eyes.

HANDLING THE YOUNG BABY

Purpose. To handle the baby with ease and with security and comfort for the baby, including a few special "holds."

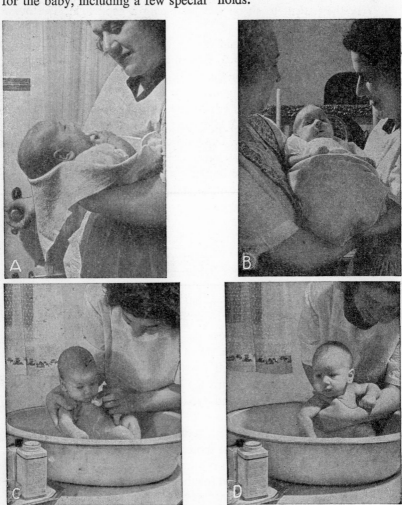

Mother needs to know how to hold baby securely and comfortably. (A) Football hold. (B) Cradle hold used in passing baby from one person to another. (C-D) For security in holding slippery baby. (C) Body hold (back). (D) Body hold (front).

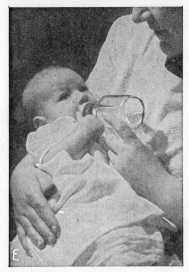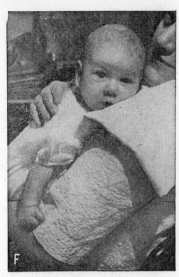

(E) Proper support for giving bottle. (F) Bubbling.

Equipment

Protected surface, such as a bed or table   Clean towel or cloth

Procedures

To Lift a Baby.

1. With one hand grasp the feet at the ankles, placing one finger between the ankles for comfort and security and raising the buttocks slightly.

2. Slip the other hand along the back and support the back and head with the fingers spread.

3. Lift gently and shift into the arms, supporting the head and back.

To Carry by the Football Hold (Allowing the Holder One Free Hand).

1. Lift the baby.

2. Swing the baby so that the baby's hip rests on the holder's hip on the same side as the arm, which together with the outspread hand supports the baby's head and shoulders securely.

To Use the Cradle Hold (for Transferring a Baby from One Person to Another).

1. Hold the baby in both arms, using the "cradle position."

2. Have the receiver hold the arms forward, slightly bent to make a "cradle."

3. Place the baby in the bend of the receiver's arms, providing a double cradle before the arms of one person are removed to give the baby a feeling of security.

To Use the Body-arm Hold (as When Giving the Baby a Tub Bath).

1. With one arm support the back of the head and shoulders, and grasp the baby's far arm at the shoulder.

2. With the other arm, support the buttocks and grasp the baby's far leg at the thigh.

3. Gently lower the baby into the water, feet first because quick motions tend to frighten the baby. Maintain a grasp of the arm during the bath.

4. Shift the arms for the hold to wash and rinse the back, reaching across the chest and grasping the baby's far arm at the shoulder, and letting the baby rest forward on the holder's arm while his back is washed and rinsed.

5. Return to the original hold, supporting the back of the head and shoulders and the buttocks, and lift the baby gently out of the tub.

To "Bubble" the Baby on the Shoulder or Lap.

SHOULDER.

1. Place a clean towel or cloth on the shoulder.

2. Lift the baby and place the baby's head against the shoulder. Allow space for breathing.

3. Support his back and head and gently rub or pat his back to help the baby release swallowed air.

LAP.

1. Place a clean cloth on the knees.

2. Place the baby face down across the knees of the holder.

3. Gently rub his back, allowing the baby to release the swallowed air.

Essential Points To Remember.

1. Support the back and head at all times.

2. Lift gently, avoiding sudden motions.

3. Provide an opportunity for the baby to release swallowed air after feeding.

4. Maintain a secure but gentle grasp when handling a baby.

CARING FOR THE BABY'S BOTTLES

Purpose. To cleanse and boil the baby's bottles and other equipment needed for giving water, fruit juice, milk, or a formula.

Equipment

Stove or other provision for boiling water

Containers for water, hot and cold

Dishpan

Soap or detergent

Bottle brush

Pencil or other blunt instrument

Extra saucepan

Nipple container with a whole lid (for the clean nipples)

Large cooking kettle

Supply of nursing bottles

Supply of nipples

Nipple covers or caps, improvised or commercial

Lifter—a large kitchen spoon, large fork, or some other lifter

Funnel

Perforated lid for a nipple container or a cloth large enough to wrap the supply of nipples

Procedure

1. Rinse the soiled bottles with *cold* water. Wash thoroughly with hot soapy water, using a brush and rinse well.

2. Rinse the nipples with cold water. Wash thoroughly with hot sudsy water, turning the nipples inside out with the eraser end of a pencil or other blunt instrument to cleanse the inside.

3. Place the bottles, nipples (either wrapped in the cloth or in the jar closed with a perforated top), lifter, and other utensils in water with the mouth of every jar and bottle under water. When preparing a formula using powdered milk, a measuring spoon, a knife for leveling the milk, and a measuring cup for liquid milk should be included.

4. Boil 5 minutes from the start of boiling.

5. Remove the articles from the pan with a lifter. Avoid touching the rims or insides of the jars and nipples with the hands. Allow to drain. Keep clean.

6. Drain the water from the nipples and cover the jar with a whole lid or remove the nipples from the cloth and place in a container; cover with a whole lid.

7. Fill the bottles with boiled water, a formula prepared according to the doctor's orders, or fruit juice, using a funnel for ease in pouring.

8. Place the nipples on the bottles:

   a. Handle the nipple at the outer lower edge to keep the nipple top clean and untouched as it is to go into the baby's mouth.

   b. Cup the index finger firmly around the base of the nipple on the far side of the mouth of the bottle to hold securely.

   c. With the other hand, pull the nipple forward, using a circular pull, and over the rim of the bottle.

   d. Place a clean cover (glass, napkin, oiled paper) over the nipple.

9. Refrigerate if a formula.

10. Warm the water or formula before feeding the baby by placing the bottle in a container of warm water.

11. Test the flow and temperature of the fluid by shaking a few drops on the inner surface of the wrist (warm to the wrist).

12. If necessary, enlarge the holes in the nipple with a needle that has been passed through a flame to clean it and heat it for ease in perforating the rubber.

Essential Points To Remember.

1. Have clean hands, apron, and area on which to work.
2. Use only clean boiled utensils.
3. Test for temperature (warm to the wrist) and flow before feeding.
4. If a formula is prepared, have the doctor's orders.
5. Keep the formula covered and cold.
6. Warm the formula before feeding; avoid giving the baby a reheated formula; dispose of any leftovers after each feeding.

MAKING SUBSTITUTE EQUIPMENT

There are many times during a short illness or in an emergency when a piece of equipment must be improvised out of the materials at hand. Serviceable and durable invalid furniture may occasionally be made at home at much less cost than if purchased. There is, however, some equipment that should be purchased, rented, or borrowed, especially for a long illness, such as a comfortable bed of the right height.

Before making, buying, or putting a piece of equipment into use, check these points:

1. Is it safe for the patient, nurse, or homemaker to use? Will there be any danger in its use to children or anyone else in the house? Will it injure the home furniture or utensils in any way?
2. Does it serve its purpose and is it durable?
3. Is it easy to keep clean?
4. Will it bring comfort to the patient and is it easy to handle?
5. Will it be less costly to make at home than to buy?
6. Are the skill and time available to make the article so that it functions safely and smoothly, looks reasonably attractive, and will last as long as the patient needs it?

Back Rest

Several types of back rests can be purchased; an improvised back rest frequently is just as good, however, and is easily made or adjusted. Some suggestions are:

1. A folded card table or a large pastry board, covered and slanted against the head of the bed and tied securely in place.

2. A washboard slipped into a pillow case with the pillow braced and tied in place.

3. Overstuffed cushions from a chair or davenport, covered and, if necessary, tied in place.

4. A large cardboard carton.

Making a Cardboard Carton Back Rest.

Purpose. To use as a back support for a bed patient when in a sitting position.

Equipment

Large cardboard carton approximately 20×20×18 inches with cover flaps
Knife

Strong cord
Cloth to cover the carton

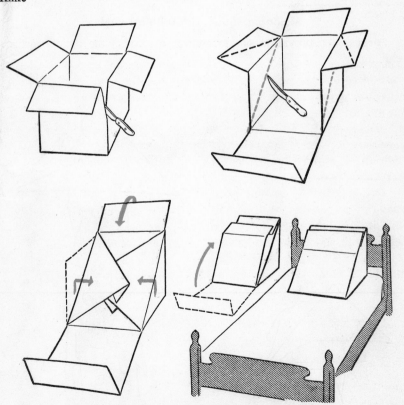

A back rest can be made from a cardboard box.

Procedure

1. Select the broad side of the carton for the front.

2. Cut down the corner at each end—from top to bottom.

3. Score the short sides of the carton diagonally from the top back to the bottom front—inner surface.

4. Bend the sides inward along the line of scoring.

5. Score and bend inward any excess of cardboard at the top or sides of the carton.

6. Bend the top flap down and bring the front side and flap up over the folded sides, scoring and bending any excess. This forms a triangular back rest.

7. Tie the back rest with a strong cord and cover for neatness and for protection of the bed and bedding.

8. Place on the bed with the slanting side toward the patient.

Making a Shawl with a Bath Towel

Purpose. To provide a shoulder cover to protect the patient against chilling.

Equipment

Large bath towel   Safety pin

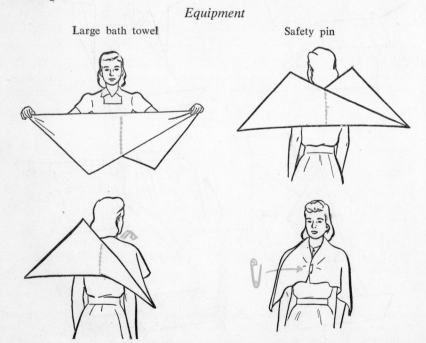

Using a large towel as a shoulder shawl.

Procedure

1. Grasp the diagonally opposite corners of the towel lengthwise and pull so that the towel is folded diagonally.

2. Locate the V that is formed by the fold and place the towel on the shoulders, bringing the V to the back of the patient's neck.

3. Bring the two points over the shoulder and pin evenly in front.

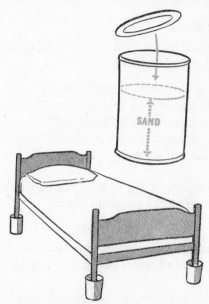

Having the bed at proper height saves energy of the home nurse.

Providing Bed Blocks

Purpose. To raise the height of the bed to a convenient working level. Three safe types of home-made bed blocks are suggested here.

Making Tin Can Blocks.

Equipment

4 large-size cans with tops which have been cut off   Sand, small pebbles, or gravel

Procedure

1. Smooth the edge of the cans for safety.

2. Fill each can about one-half full of sand or pebbles. All cans must be filled to the same level.

3. Drop the top of the can on top of the sand.

4. Place a can under each leg of the bed after removing the caster.

Using Broad-based Cinder Blocks.

1. Remove the casters.

2. Place one block under each leg of the bed—all should be the same height.

Making Wooden Blocks.

These can be made at the local lumber yard or in the manual training department of the high school.

Equipment and Procedure

1. Select four pieces of hard lumber that will not crack or split, all of equal size (approximately $8 \times 8 \times 12$ inches).

2. Bore a hole 6 inches deep (or one-half of the depth) and large enough to admit the bed leg without the caster in the center of one end of each block.

3. Place the bed legs in the block holes and make sure the bed is well steadied and the blocks are firmly placed.

Bed Table

Purpose. To provide a convenient table space for the bed patient who is able to sit up to eat or write, play cards, and carry on other similar activities.

Adjustable tables to be used by bed patients may be purchased; some are placed on the bed; others have a floor stand with a table surface on an adjustable arm that swings into the desired position over the bed.

One simple improvisation for a single bed is the use of an ironing board on a stand with the board swung across the bed, or the plain board resting on the straight backs or between the slats of two chairs, one on either side of the bed.

Making and Placing a Cardboard Carton Bed Table
For a Patient Who Can Sit Up

Equipment

Clean, heavy cardboard carton, approximately $24 \times 10 \times 12$ inches

Knife

Suitable cover

Procedure

1. Remove all the top covers.

2. Cut out the curved portions of the long sides to allow the "table"

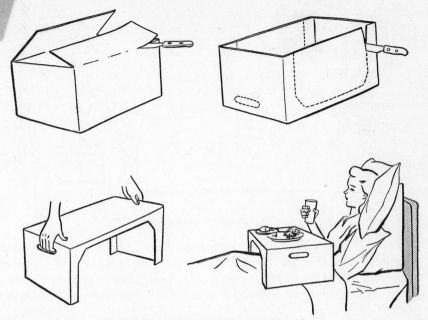

Making a cardboard carton bed table.

to fit comfortably over the patient's thighs. Always hold the knife blade away from the body when cutting.

3. Cut small openings in the upper portion of the short ends—these allow easy handling of the table.

4. Cover—this may be cloth, paint, or wallpaper.

5. Place on the bed—free the bedding on either side of the patient's thighs to permit looseness over the thighs; adjust the table to a comfortable level for the patient's use. With the bedding loose, the patient can move and adjust to a comfortable position more easily and there is less danger of upsetting the articles on the table.

An orange crate or soap box can be used in the same way as the cardboard carton. An attractive cretonne or oilcloth cover can be made with pockets on the sides for convenient storage space for spectacles, writing materials, and other articles that need to be within easy reach.

Bed Cradle

Purpose. To keep the weight of the bed clothes off the patient, this may include the entire body or an affected part.

Such a cradle may be purchased or it may be made at home from a

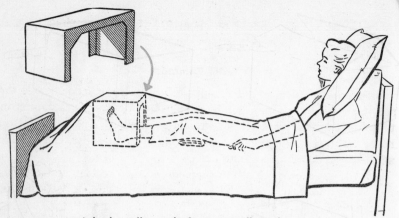

A bed cradle made from a cardboard carton.

lightweight wooden box, crate, or cardboard carton. This is made in the same manner as the cardboard table. The size of the carton will depend upon the part of the body to be protected. A soft piece of flannel or a hot water bag well wrapped should be provided if extra warmth is needed.

Providing Toe Space for the Bed Patient

To provide toe space at the foot of the bed, make a double pleat lengthwise with the sheet and blanket together. Tuck in loosely at the foot and sides. (*See* p. 148.)

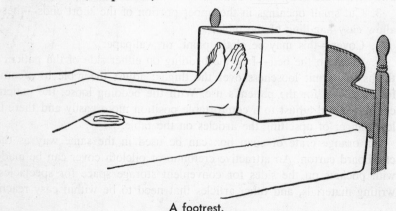

A footrest.

Providing a Footrest

A cardboard carton (approximately $14 \times 12 \times 9$ inches) or other suitable support may be used. Adjust the footrest securely at the foot of the bed. The support should be about 2 inches higher than the toes to keep the covers from pressing on the toes.

A Toilet Commode

Sometimes the doctor will permit the use of a commode beside the bed. A commode may be made by placing a slop jar under a cut-out in the seat of a low, comfortable, straight-back chair. A covered lid on hinges will make the commode serviceable as a chair also, and a ruffle attached will make it more attractive.

It is very important that the commode and jar be kept scrupulously clean at all times to avoid unpleasant odors. A commode may also be purchased or rented.

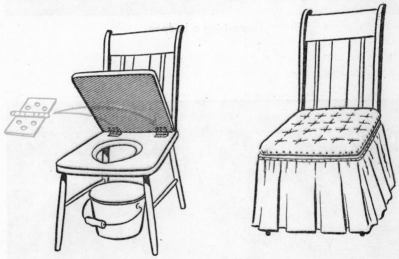

Using a chair to improvise a commode.

Making an Improvised Bedpan and Urinal

Purpose. To receive the bed patient's body wastes such as urine and bowel movements when the patient is unable to go to the toilet.

An improvised bedpan may be made if a commercial bedpan cannot be obtained.

Equipment

Cardboard carton approximately
 14×12×6 inches
Knife

Basin
Newspapers

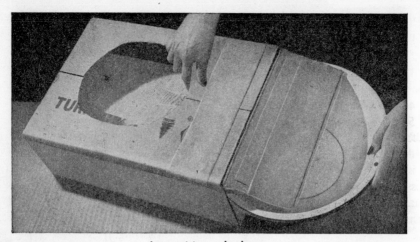

Improvising a bedpan.

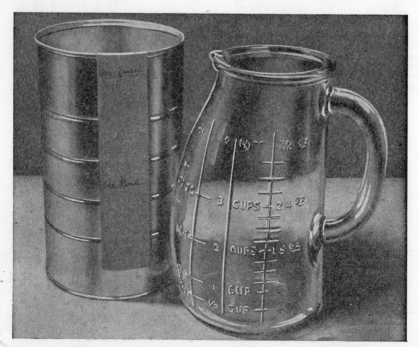

An improvised (left) and a commercial urinal (right).

Procedure

1. Select one side for the bottom of the box. Be sure it is firm.
2. Leave one end open.
3. Cut an oval opening for the seat on the top surface of the box about 3 or 4 inches from the closed end.
4. Insert the basin under the opening.
5. Have the basin as close to the top of the box as possible. (Prop with newspapers or other material.)

A urinal is a cuplike or bottle-shaped vessel to receive urine only. It is essential for men and boys. Substitutes for use in a temporary illness may be a glass jar, a tin can with its rough edges smoothed, or a quart measure; the last is useful if the doctor wishes the urine measured. Whatever article is used, it must be labeled clearly and kept for this use alone; when no longer needed, it must be thoroughly cleansed or discarded.

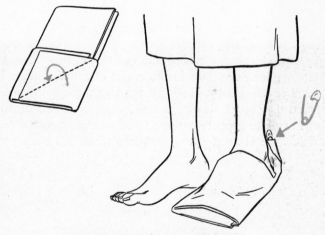

Newspaper bedroom slippers.

Making a Paper Slipper or Scuffs

Purpose. To provide protection for the feet when the patient is out of bed.

Equipment

2 double sheets of newspaper *or* heavy brown paper

2 safety pins or needle and thread

Procedure

1. Proceed as in the procedure for making a newspaper bag (p. 139) up to step 6.
2. Turn the loose end of the cuff inside to form a triangle, making the sole of the slipper.
3. Turn the slipper over.
4. Slip the hand in the cuff to raise the toe of the slipper.
5. Make a heel by pinning or stitching the back of the slipper.
6. Stitch the sole for further strength if desired.

Providing Support and Protection for Pressure Areas Such as the Elbow, Heel, Ear, Shoulder, or End of the Spine

Areas of the bed patient's body that often become tender because of continued pressure may be relieved and a sore prevented by placing a soft support under the part and lightly bandaging it in place. Cotton pads larger than the affected part furnish a good, smooth support. Air-foam or lamb's wool pads may also be used.

For temporary support, rings or "donuts" made of soft material are often used. A large ring suitable for use at the end of the spine can be made by stuffing a long stocking with cotton and tying the toe and top together; by punching a hole in the center of a thick square of cotton batting and covering it by winding a bandage through the hole, around and around the cotton, shaping it into a ring; or from foam rubber. A cut-out is made to support the part to be protected; then a center hole smaller than the affected part is cut, into which the bony prominence is fitted.

Making a Stocking "Donut."

Equipment

A clean stocking, preferably of cotton
or soft wool for a more
substantial support

Procedure

1. Turn the stocking inside out so that the smooth side of the seam will be next to the skin.
2. Beginning at the hem or top, roll firmly over and over toward the outside all the way, including the toe.
3. Use under the affected part—the heel, elbow, ear, or some other part of the body.

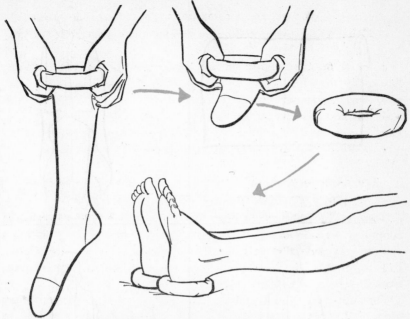

Using a stocking to make a "donut" support.

Making a Blanket Bathrobe

Purpose. To provide warmth and protection for the patient when up and about.

When a patient has been in bed for some time, getting up becomes quite an occasion. The home nurse will need to see that the patient does not become chilled and that he is comfortably protected. The patient will need some type of bath robe and in the event he has none, one can be easily improvised by using a blanket.

Equipment

Ordinary single blanket — the weight to be determined by the temperature—long enough to cover the patient's legs and ankles

3 safety pins

Procedure

1. Make a collar along the length of the blanket—the width of the collar depends upon the size of the patient and the size of the blanket.

2. Adjust on the patient's shoulders, centering the collar at the back

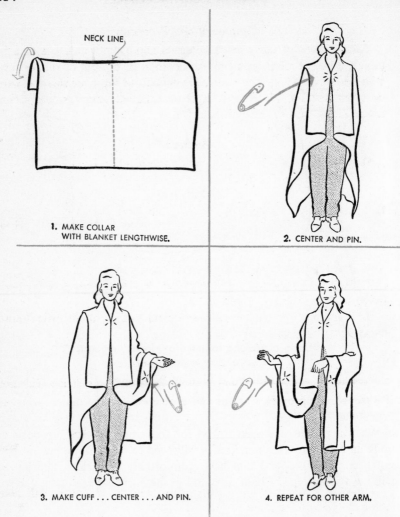

1. MAKE COLLAR WITH BLANKET LENGTHWISE.

2. CENTER AND PIN.

3. MAKE CUFF . . . CENTER . . . AND PIN.

4. REPEAT FOR OTHER ARM.

Making a blanket robe.

of the patient's neck, and bring the blanket around to the front and pin.

3. Make sleeves, centering the width of the blanket; place at the wrist; turn back the cuff and pin.

Door Silencer

Purpose. To silence the click of the door latch and make it easier to open and close the sickroom door quietly.

Equipment and Procedure

Take a piece of fairly heavy material about 3×5 inches with a tape (about 6 inches long) sewed to each corner, or a piece of rubber tubing with holes cut at either end and long enough to slip over the doorknobs, or an old stocking. Place the silencer over the latch and fasten it securely to the doorknobs.

Bedpad

Purpose. To provide protection for the bedding.

Equipment

12 thicknesses of newspaper

Cloth large enough to extend about 6 inches beyond paper on all sides

Procedure

1. Place the papers in the center of the cloth.
2. Make an envelope by folding the cloth over the edges of the paper; fasten at the corners.
3. When placing, put the cloth side next to the patient; when removing, fold with the cloth side in.

Cotton Swab or Applicator

Purpose. To be used to apply medication and to cleanse such areas as wounds or the mouth of a helpless patient.

Equipment

Absorbent cotton   Sticks—toothpicks or other   Water

Procedure

1. Select a small piece of cotton; the amount of cotton will determine the size of the swab.
2. Wet the stick so that the cotton will adhere to it.
3. Place the moist end in the center of the cotton to cover the end of the stick for protection and the patient's comfort.
4. Roll the stick, holding the cotton firmly at the bottom of the swab.
5. Shape.

Essential Points To Remember.
1. Cover the tip.
2. Be sure the cotton is wrapped securely.
3. Use only once.

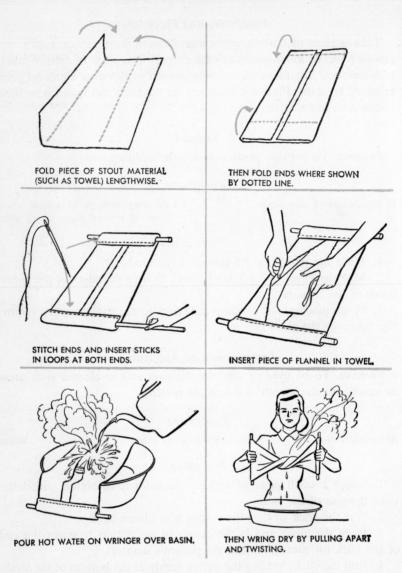

FOLD PIECE OF STOUT MATERIAL
(SUCH AS TOWEL) LENGTHWISE.

THEN FOLD ENDS WHERE SHOWN
BY DOTTED LINE.

STITCH ENDS AND INSERT STICKS
IN LOOPS AT BOTH ENDS.

INSERT PIECE OF FLANNEL IN TOWEL.

POUR HOT WATER ON WRINGER OVER BASIN.

THEN WRING DRY BY PULLING APART
AND TWISTING.

How to make a wringer for hot moist compress.

Compress or Stupe Wringer

Purpose. To use in wringing "dry" large, hot, moist compresses without harming the hands or allowing the compress to cool.

Equipment and Procedure

Take a piece of strong cloth long enough to extend well over the sides of the basin to be used and wide enough to hold the compress (usually about 18×18 inches) and 2 stout sticks, e.g., pieces of broom handle (about 10 inches long).

Fold the edges toward the center of the cloth; hem the ends; slip the sticks through the hems.

Chart of Selected Communicable Diseases

To prevent the spread of infection, any person suspected of having a communicable disease should be kept away from others. Measures for the control of communicable diseases are established either by law or regulation in the various states and communities. As these may vary, each individual should keep in touch with the local health authorities and be responsible for coöperating with them in preventing the spread of disease.

Disease	How Spread	Prevention	How Long from Exposure to Onset	Common Symptoms	How Long Communicable	Some Possible Complications
Chickenpox	Directly from person to person; indirectly through articles freshly soiled by discharges from the skin and mucous membrane of infected persons.	No immunization available; avoid exposure; one attack usually gives immunity.	2 to 3 weeks.	Small reddish pimples or blisters; usually more abundant on the covered than the exposed parts of the body, which become itchy; slight fever.	Probably not more than 1 day before or more than 6 days after pimples first appear; highly communicable during the early stages.	Rarely, the skin eruptions may become infected.
Common cold	Contact with discharges from the nose and throat; directly from person to person; indirectly through articles freshly soiled by discharges.	No specific prevention; maintain body resistance and avoid chilling and exposure to illness.	12 to 72 hours.	Tickling, dry sensation in the throat; slight fever; chilliness; sick feeling; cough and runny nose.	Usually limited to the early stage of the disease.	Bronchitis, laryngitis, pneumonia, middle ear infection in children.
Diphtheria	Contact with discharges from the nose and throat or other infected membranes; by carriers as well as by sick persons; milk may carry the germs of the disease.	Immunization in infancy, with reinforcing doses periodically; adults exposed to infection should be given a Schick test to determine susceptibility before immunization; second at-	2 to 5 days, sometimes longer.	Inflammation of the tonsils, throat, and nose, with grayish white patches; fever.	Until the germs have disappeared as shown by tests; usually 2 weeks or less.	Damage to the heart and throat muscles.

Disease	How Spread	Prevention	Incubation Period	Symptoms	Period Communicable	Complications
	charges from the bowels of infected persons; contaminated food and water; flies.	avoidance of known sources; personal cleanliness; repeated attacks possible.	days.		contain the infecting agent as checked by laboratory tests; sometimes weeks.	
German measles (Rubella)	Contact with discharges from the throat and mouth; easily communicable.	No immunization; second attacks rare; especially important to guard women in early pregnancy against exposure.	10 to 21 days.	Slight cold followed by a red rash on the face and body; small, beady lumps behind the ears; slight fever (frequently confused with scarlet fever).	From onset and for at least 4 days, possibly 7.	None usually; serious for women during early pregnancy as it may result in a defect of the baby if the mother contracts measles during early pregnancy.
Gonorrhea	Contact with fresh discharges from the genital tract of infected persons or from other infected areas such as the eyes; most frequently through sexual intercourse.	No immunization; avoidance of contact; medicine put in the eyes of newborn babies; one attack does not confer immunity.	1 to 14 days; usually 3 to 5 days.	A pus discharge from a mucous membrane of the genital tract or of the eyes.	As long as the germ appears in the discharges, as checked by laboratory tests.	Arthritis, sterility, infection of the eyes of the newborn.
Impetigo	Contact with moist discharges from sores on the skin; possibly nose and throat discharges.	No immunization; reinfections possible.	Perhaps 2 to 5 days.	Running sores on the face and hands or body, later showing crusts.	As long as the sores are unhealed.	Occasional infection of the sores.
Infantile paralysis (Poliomyelitis)	Contact with the nose, throat, and bowel discharges of infected persons or carriers.	No immunization available; adults have more immunity than children; one attack usually confers immunity.	Usually 7 to 14 days (may be from 3 to 35 days).	Many cases not recognized; fever, headache, drowsiness, stiff neck and back, and irritability.	Not exactly known, probably the later part of the incubation period and the first week of acute illness.	Paralysis of the affected parts of the body.

CHART OF SELECTED COMMUNICABLE DISEASES (Continued)

Disease	How Spread	Prevention	How Long from Exposure to Onset	Common Symptoms	How Long Communicable	Some Possible Complications
Influenza	Contact with discharges from the nose and mouth and articles freshly soiled with discharges.	Ask the doctor about immunization; repeated attacks are possible.	24 to 72 hours.	Sudden onset; fever, aching limbs and back, runny nose, sore throat, bronchitis, and prostration.	Uncertain.	Pneumonia.
Measles	Contact with discharges of the nose and throat; easily spread.	No immunization but attack may be lightened or prevented in children exposed to measles if immune serum globulin is given; babies of immune mothers are usually immune for the first few months of life; one attack usually confers immunity.	Usually about 10 days from exposure to onset of the fever; 13 to 15 days to the appearance of the rash; as long as 21 days if immune serum globulin has been given.	Fever, runny eyes and nose, eruption in the mouth, followed by rash; branny peeling of the skin during convalescence.	During the period of runny eyes and nose, usually about 9 days (from 4 days before to 5 days after the rash appears).	Inflammation of the middle ear, pneumonia.
Epidemic meningitis	Contact with discharges of the nose and throat; carriers.	No immunization; avoid contact, droplet infection, and overcrowding; stress personal cleanliness.	2 to 10 days; usually 7 days.	Usually a sudden onset; fever, headache, nausea, and vomiting; rash occasionally; dizziness, stiff neck, and delirium.	Until the germs disappear from the discharges, as checked by laboratory tests.	Spread of the infection to the tissue of the brain.

	How Spread	Prevention	Incubation Period	Symptoms	Communicable Period	Complications
Mumps	Contact with the saliva of infected persons.	No immunization; second attacks have been known but are rare.	12 to 26 days; usually 18 days.	Fever, swelling of the salivary glands in the cheeks and under the tongue.	From 1 to 2 days before the symptoms appear until swelling of the glands has disappeared.	Inflammation of the ovaries or testicles in persons past puberty.
Rheumatic* fever	Unknown.	No immunization; disease recurs.	Unknown; it may be several days to 8 weeks after infection before the symptoms appear; the average is 3 weeks.	Fever, joint and muscle pains; sometimes nosebleed; rapid pulse and loss of appetite; may begin slowly.	See Footnote.	Serious damage to the heart.
Ringworm	Contact with the sores, discharges from the sores, or clothing in contact with the sores; contact with infected cats or dogs.	No immunization; repeated attacks common.	Not known.	Round, scaly patches on the scalp or body; likely to appear on the feet, and between the toes as well; itching.	As long as the fungus or spores remain around the sores.	Occasional secondary infection of the sores.
Scabies	Contact with an infected person or articles in contact with an infected person.	Avoid contact; repeated infestation common.	24 to 48 hours.	"Burrows" or lines of sores; severe itching, particularly between the fingers.	Until the itch mite and eggs are destroyed.	Occasional infection of the sores.

* Not communicable. The infection that has preceded this disease is communicable but has usually subsided by the time the symptoms of rheumatic fever appear.

CHART OF SELECTED COMMUNICABLE DISEASES *(Continued)*

Disease	How Spread	Prevention	How Long from Exposure to Onset	Common Symptoms	How Long Communicable	Some Possible Complications
Scarlet† fever	Contact with discharges of the nose, throat, or ears of infected person; carriers; contaminated milk or other foods.	No immunization; pasteurization of milk; avoidance of contact with ill persons.	1 to 5 days.	Sore, inflamed throat; strawberry tongue; fever, nausea, and vomiting; later a rash, usually beginning on the neck and chest.	Not known; 2 weeks at least.	Inflammation of the middle ear; damage to the heart and kidneys; rheumatic fever.
Smallpox	Contact with nose and throat discharges and sores on the bodies of patients.	Vaccination gives protection if the rules are followed; one attack usually prevents another.	7 to 16 days, occasionally longer; commonly 12 days.	Fever and a general feeling of illness, followed by the eruption 1 to 5 days later; the crusts fall off in 10 to 40 days; the disease may vary from mild to very severe with a high death rate.	From the first symptom to the disappearance of the crusts of the eruption; most communicable in the early stages of the illness.	Pitting of the skin, occasional blindness, bronchitis, ear infection.
Syphilis	Contact with discharge from known sores or those hidden on the mucous membrane and skin; usually contracted through sexual intercourse; blood of infected persons.	No immunization; one attack does *not* prevent another.	10 days to 3 weeks or longer.	Sore at the point of contact, which will heal but may recur during the next 5 years after infection; in congenital syphilis, only the late manifestations, such as those listed under complications, occur.	From onset and, if untreated, up to 5 years.	Damage to the heart and central nervous system, including the brain, unless treated early.

† The germ causing scarlet fever, hemolytic streptococci, may also cause other diseases such as streptococcal sore throat, erysipelas,

	How spread	Prevention	Incubation period	Symptoms	Period communicable	Complications
Tetanus	Infected soil, street dust, and animal feces introduced through a break in the skin, especially through puncture wounds such as those made by nails.	Tetanus toxoid—requires reinforcing at certain intervals; one attack does not protect; antitoxin is given in the presence of a suspected wound.	4 days to 3 weeks.	Painful muscular movements; pain in the cheek or neck muscles on chewing and swallowing; infection of the umbilical cord in the newborn.	Not passed on to another person.	Rare under proper treatment and prevention; highly fatal if not treated promptly.
Tuberculosis, pulmonary	Contact with the discharges of the nose and throat from an "active" tuberculous case; occasionally by milk from tuberculous cattle.	No immunization; one attack does *not* prevent another; pasteurization of milk; killing of tuberculous cattle.	Variable; probably not less than 1 month and possibly longer.	Usually no noticeable symptoms until the disease is moderately advanced; then fatigue, loss of weight, chronic cough, loss of appetite, afternoon rise in temperature.	For the duration of the active state of the disease as shown by tests and x-ray.	Meningitis, miliary (general) tuberculosis.
Typhoid fever	Contact with infected feces and urine; contaminated water or food, especially milk.	Typhoid vaccine gives immunity for about 2 years; one attack usually prevents another.	3 to 38 days; usually 7 to 14 days.	Fever, headache, diarrhea, and "stomach-ache"; later "rose spots" on the trunk.	As long as the typhoid germs appear in the discharges from the bowels as checked by laboratory tests.	Hemorrhage, bronchitis, pneumonia.
Undulant fever (Brucellosis)	Contact with infected animals; milk of infected animals.	No immunization; boiling or pasteurization of milk.	6 to 30 days or more.	Slow onset; irregular fever, sweating, chills, and pain in the joints and muscles.	Not communicable from man to man.	Disease may be prolonged through months and years.

CHART OF SELECTED COMMUNICABLE DISEASES (*Continued*)

Disease	How Spread	Prevention	How Long from Exposure to Onset	Common Symptoms	How Long Communicable	Some Possible Complications
Whooping cough	Contact with infected discharges of the nose and throat.	Immunization giving considerable protection is available; one attack usually prevents another; reinforcing doses of vaccine may be advisable within a year and at 2 or 3 years of age.	7 to 21 days.	Typical "whooping" cough develops from ordinary cough in 1 to 2 weeks; suspect any cough when the disease is known to be present in the neighborhood.	From onset to 3 weeks.	Bronchitis, bronchial pneumonia; frequently fatal to young babies.

SUPPLEMENTARY READING*

BOOKS AND PAMPHLETS

American National Red Cross: *First Aid Textbook,* rev. ed., Philadelphia, The Blakiston Company, 1945. Cloth $1, paper 60 cents.

Armstrong, Donald B., and Hallock, Grace T.: *What To Do Till the Doctor Comes,* New York, Simon and Schuster, 1943. $1.50.

Beardwood, Joseph T., and Kelly, Herbert T.: *Simplified Diabetic Management,* 5th ed., Philadelphia, J. B. Lippincott Co., 1947. $2.50.

Boyd, Neva L.: *Hospital and Bedside Games,* rev. ed., Chicago, H. T. Fitzsimons Co., Inc., 1945. $1.

Colcord, Joanna C.: *Your Community; Its Provision for Health, Education, Safety and Welfare,* rev. by Donald S. Howard, New York, Russell Sage Foundation, 1947. $1.50.

Cooper, Lenna F., and others: *Nutrition in Health and Disease,* 11th ed., rev., Philadelphia, J. B. Lippincott Co., 1950.

Dakin, Florence, and Thompson, Ella M.: *Simplified Nursing,* 4th ed., Philadelphia, J. B. Lippincott Co., 1941. $3.

Diehl, Harold S.: *Healthful Living,* new 3d ed., New York, McGraw-Hill Book Co., 1949. $4.50.

Faegre, Marion L., and Anderson, John E.: *Child Care and Training,* 7th ed. rev., Minneapolis, University of Minnesota Press, 1947. $3.25.

Fishbein, Morris: *Common Ailments of Man,* Garden City, N. Y., Garden City Publishing Co., 1945. $1.

Gesell, Arnold: *How a Baby Grows: A Story in Pictures,* New York, Paul B. Hoeber, Inc., 1945. $2.

Gesell, Arnold, and Ilg, Frances L.: *The Child from Five to Ten,* New York, Paul B. Hoeber, Inc., 1946. $4.50.

Kawin, Ethel: *The Wise Choice of Toys,* rev. ed., Chicago, University of Chicago Press, 1938. $2.50.

Monsch, Helen, and Harper, M. K.: *Feeding Babies and Their Family,* New York, John Wiley & Sons, Inc., 1943. $3.50.

National Bureau of Standards: *Safety for the Household,* Circular No. 463, Washington, D. C., U. S. Government Printing Office, 1948. 75 cents.

New York Academy of Medicine, Committee on Public Health Relations: *Directory of Convalescent Homes in the United States,* White Plains, N. Y., The Burke Foundation, 1947. 50 cents.

---

* This is only a suggested list of the many references available.

Norlin, Elinor, and Donaldson, Bessie M.: *Everyday Nursing for the Everyday Home,* New York, The Macmillan Co., 1942. $2.75.

Olson, Lyla M.: *Improvised Equipment in the Home Care of the Sick,* 4th ed., Philadelphia, W. B. Saunders Co., 1947. $1.50.

Porter, Edna (Comp.): *Community Wise,* New York, Woman's Press, 1947. 75 cents.

Preston, George Heinrichs: *Psychiatry for the Curious,* New York, Rinehart & Co., Inc., 1940. $2.

Rand, Winifred, and others: *The Growth and Development of the Young Child,* 4th ed., Philadelphia, W. B. Saunders Co., 1946. $3.50.

Rose, Mary Swartz: *Feeding the Family,* 4th ed., New York, The Macmillan Co., 1940. $4.25.

Spock, Benjamin: *The Common Sense Book of Baby and Child Care,* New York, Duell, Sloan & Pearce, 1946. $3.

Spock, Benjamin: *The Pocket Book of Baby and Child Care,* New York, Pocketbooks, Inc., 1945. 35 cents.

Stern, Edith M., and Corcoran, Mary E.: *The Attendant's Guide,* New York, The Commonwealth Fund, 1945. 50 cents.

Stern, Edith M., and Hamilton, Samuel W.: *Mental Illness: A Guide for the Family,* rev. ed., New York, The Commonwealth Fund, 1945. $1.

Stieglitz, Edward J.: *The Second Forty Years,* Philadelphia, J. B. Lippincott Co., 1946. $3.

Todd, Ramona L., and Freeman, Ruth B.: *Health Care of the Family,* Philadelphia, W. B. Saunders Co., 1946. $3.50.

U.S. Department of Agriculture: *Family Fare,* Home and Garden Bulletin No. 1, Washington, D.C., U.S. Government Printing Office, 1950. 25 cents.

Vaughan, Warren T.: *Primer of Allergy,* rev. by J. Harvey Black, 3d. ed., St. Louis, C. V. Mosby Co., 1950. $3.50.

Wilkins, Walter, and Boyd, French: *Nutrition for You,* 2d ed., Jacksonville, Fla. (P.O. Box 210), 1947. 20 cents.

PERIODICALS

Child Study: Published quarterly by the Child Study Association, 132 East 74th St., New York 21, N.Y. Subscription price $2.25.

National Parent-Teacher: Published monthly by the National Parent-Teacher, Inc., 600 South Michigan Blvd., Chicago 5, Ill. Subscription price $1.

Today's Health: Published monthly by the American Medical Association, 535 North Dearborn St., Chicago 10, Ill. Subscription price $2.50.

SOURCES OF ADDITIONAL MATERIAL

(Valuable *current* information on almost every topic discussed in this book is available from most of the local health and education departments and from many other organizations—free upon request or at a nominal cost. Be specific when requesting material.)

American Cancer Society, Inc., 47 Beaver St., New York 4, N.Y. (Distribution of all materials is handled by the division offices.)

American Dental Association, 222 East Superior St., Chicago 11, Ill.

American Medical Association, 535 North Dearborn St., Chicago 10, Ill.

American Occupational Therapy Association, 33 West 42d St., New York 18, N.Y.

American Social Hygiene Association, 1790 Broadway, New York 19, N.Y.

Children's Bureau, Federal Security Agency, Washington 25, D.C.

Health departments—state, county, and city

Joint Orthopedic Nursing Advisory Service, 1790 Broadway, New York 19, N.Y.

Maternity Center Association, 654 Madison Ave., New York 21, N.Y.

National Committee for Mental Hygiene, Inc., 1790 Broadway, New York 19, N.Y.

National Foundation for Infantile Paralysis, 120 Broadway, New York, N.Y.

National Safety Council, Inc., 20 North Wacker Drive, Chicago 6, Ill.

National Society for Crippled Children and Adults, Inc., 11 South LaSalle St., Chicago 3, Ill.

National Society for the Prevention of Blindness, Inc., 1790 Broadway, New York 19, N.Y.

National Tuberculosis Association, 1790 Broadway, New York 19, N.Y.

Nursing associations—state and county

Office of Education, Federal Security Agency, Washington 25, D.C.

Public Affairs Committee, Inc., 22 East 38th St., New York 16, N.Y.

Public Health Service, Federal Security Agency, Washington 25, D.C.

U.S. Department of Agriculture, Washington 25, D.C.

SOURCES OF ADDITIONAL MATERIAL

The following sources will provide materials for further information on the topics discussed.

American Cancer Society, Inc., 47 Beaver Street, New York 4, N.Y.

American Dental Association, 222 East Superior Street, Chicago 11, Ill.

American Medical Association, 535 North Dearborn Street, Chicago 10, Ill.

American Occupational Therapy Association, ... West ....., ...

American Social Hygiene Association, 1790 Broadway, New York 19, N.Y.

Children's Bureau, Federal Security Agency, Washington 25, D.C. and state departments—state, county, and city.

Joint Orthopedic Nursing Advisory Service, 1790 Broadway, New York 19, N.Y.

Maternity Center Association, 654 Madison Ave., New York 21, N.Y.

National Committee for Mental Hygiene, Inc., 1790 Broadway, New York 19, N.Y.

National Foundation for Infantile Paralysis, 120 Broadway, New York, N.Y.

National Safety Council, Inc., 20 North Wacker Drive, Chicago 6, Ill.

National Society for Crippled Children and Adults, Inc., 11 South LaSalle St., Chicago 3, Ill.

National Society for the Prevention of Blindness, Inc., 1790 Broadway, New York 19, N.Y.

National Tuberculosis Association, 1790 Broadway, New York 19, N.Y.

Nursing organizations—state and county.

Office of Education, Federal Security Agency, Washington 25, D.C.

Public Affairs Committee, Inc., 22 East 38th St., New York 16, N.Y.

Public Health Service, Federal Security Agency, Washington 25, D.C.

U.S. Department of Agriculture, Washington 25, D.C.

INDEX

Abdominal pain, acute
    as symptom, 17
    what to do, 95
Accidents (For specific measures, *see*
        Emergencies, how to meet)
    general procedure, 88
    prevention of, 133
Adolescence, years of
    development, variation in, 113
    problems, how to meet,
        113–114
Aging and chronically ill
    aging process, nature of, 73
    changes, mental, 75
    diversions, 81
    food for, 64–65
    home nurse, points for in care,
        79–82
    old age, planning for, 73–74
    special needs of, 77–79
    what to tell doctor, 84
Ambulance, how to call, 26
Appetite, in illness, 14–15
Appliances, special, use of, 83
Applications
    cold, how to give, 186–187
    hot, how to give, 181–186

Baby, emergency birth of
    care following, 99–101
    preparation for, 99
    first year emotional needs,
        108–109
    food, 107
    growth, 108
    how to handle, 198–200
    premature, care of, 101
    sleep, 107, 109
    training, 109
Baby bottles, how to care for,
    200–202
Back rest, how to make, 202–204

Back rub, how to give, 160–161
Bath
    in bed, how to give, 156–160
    tub, how to give, 162
Bathrobe, blanket, how to make,
    213–214
Bed, for patient,
    bedspread, 43
    bedstead and springs, 40–41
    blankets, 42–43
    mattress, 41
    pillows, 42
    protection, additional, 42
    sheets, 41
Bed blocks, how to make, 205–206
Bed cradle, how to make, 207–208
Bed linen, how to change
    with patient in bed, 149–151
    without patient in bed, 147–149
Bedpad, how to make, 215
Bedpan and urinal
    how to cleanse, 69
    how to give, 162–164
    how to improvise, 209–211
Bed sores, prevention of, 46–47
Bed table, how to make, 206–207
Birth (*see* Baby, emergency birth of)
Bites, how to treat
    dog and cat, 96
    snake, poisonous, 96
    tick, 96–97
Bleeding, what to do for
    internal, 90–91
    nosebleed, 91
Bowel movements, 19–20
Burns and scalds, how to treat,
    91–92

Carrier, communicable disease, 6,
    8–10
Cesspools, danger of, 131–132
Chest pain, 17

229

NOTES

NOTES

1 rise & fall of chest
is , /——

18 Count normal
1 min ' average

68 pulse

NOTES

NOTES

NOTES

NOTES

NOTES

NOTES

NOTES

NOTES